Crystal B.

CW00348036

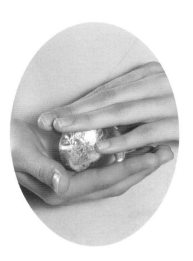

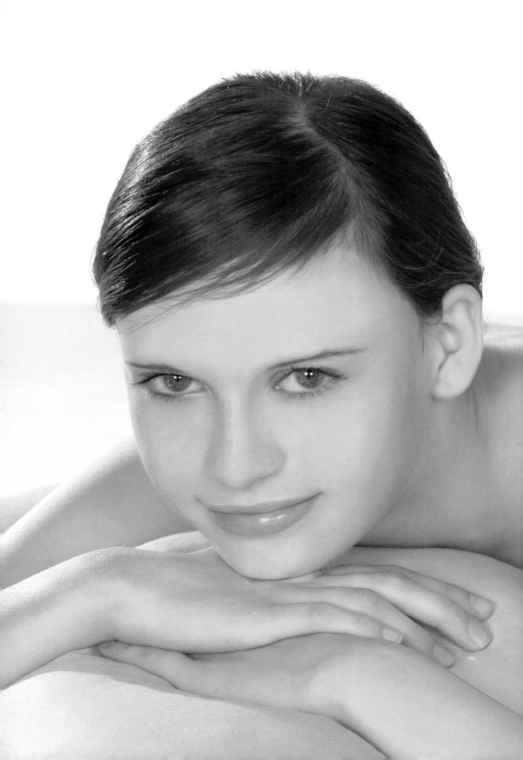

Monika Grundmann

Crystal Balance

A step-by-step guide to beauty and
health through crystal massage

Photography by
Ines Blersch

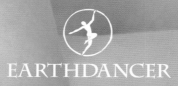

EARTHDANCER

A FINDHORN PRESS IMPRINT

Contents

Introduction by Michael Gienger 7

Crystal Balance 10

How can beauty be achieved
  through touch? 13
How did Crystal Balance originate? 16
Do you need massage oils
  to perform Crystal Balance? 17
Combining crystals and oils 18
  Serenity 19
  Security 19
  Regeneration 20
  Anti-stress 20
  Joy of Life 20
  In the Flow 21
  Fountain of Youth 21
Warm and cool crystals 23
  What is the best method of
    warming the crystals? 24
Creating the right atmosphere 25
Choosing crystals 26
  Relaxation 27
  Releasing stress and tension 28
  Achieving balance 28
  Regeneration 28
  Increasing energy levels 29
  Staying calm 29

Protection and boundaries 30
Lifting depression 30
Detoxing and purifying 30
Stimulating lymphatic flow 31
Improving circulation 31
Improving your skin 32
Exercises 33
Crystal Balance – the treatment sequence 37

Crystal Balance –
the techniques 38

Preparation 40
Protection 41
Take the weight off her shoulders 42
A grounding foot massage 53
Get to know each other better 58
Reveal the true beauty 63
Feel free! 72
Warm sun in your tummy 74
Back on your feet 79

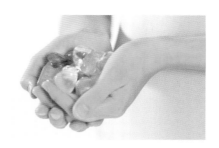

**Crystals for beauty –
the facts   86**

The aim of Crystal Balance   88

Agate   89
Amazonite   89
Amber   89
Amethyst   89
Aquamarine   90
Aventurine   90
Blue Quartz   90
Calcite, orange   91
Chalcedony, blue   91
Chrysocolla   91
Chrysoprase   91
Citrine   92
Dumortierite   92
Emerald   92
Epidote   92
Fluorite   93
Halite   93
Heliotrope   93
Hematite   94
Jasper, red   94
Kabamba Jasper   94
Magnesite   95
Malachite   95
Mookaite   95

Moonstone   95
Moss Agate   96
Nephrite   96
Obsidian   96
Ocean Agate (Ocean Jasper)   97
Petrified Wood   97
Prase   97
Rhodonite   97
Rock Crystal   98
Rose Quartz   98
Ruby-Kyanite-Fuchsite   98
Serpentine   98
Smoky Quartz   99
Sodalite   99
Sunstone   99
Tiger Iron   99
Topaz   100
Tourmaline, black (Schorl)   100
Tourmaline, green (Verdelite)   100
Tourmalinated Quartz   101
Zoisite with Ruby   101

Cleansing and care   102

The author   104
Acknowledgements   105
Addresses   106
Bibliography   108

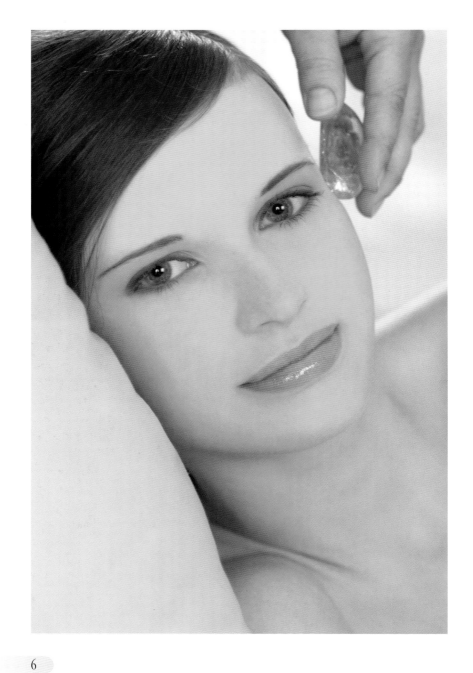

Introduction

by Michael Gienger

Beauty is an expression of wellbeing, joie de vivre and inner harmony. This is not to say that beautiful people are never sad or miserable, but rather that a feeling of wellbeing and harmony helps the beauty that is inside us all to blossom and unfold. It is the reason that massage and treatments for wellbeing are said to 'make us beautiful' and bring our real, deep, inner beauty to light.

Holistic beauty therapist Monika Grundmann knows just how to awaken this inner beauty. She regards massage, or the 'art of touching' (from the Arabic *massa*, to touch), as an important aid to achieving physical, emotional and spiritual wellbeing.

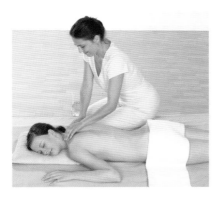

This is because body, mind and spirit are all connected, so anything that has a positive effect on the physical body will also have a positive effect on both mind and spirit. 'Of course, I cannot change the lives of my clients,' she says, 'but after a really effective massage, they feel able to approach life differently, in spite of all its problems, stresses and strains. And beauty nourishes beauty — if we feel and experience beauty, we see beauty and become beautiful too.'

And when it comes to massages, Monika's are beautiful indeed! She works with the confidence and assurance that come from many years of experience and every movement is well-judged and precise. While working as a self-employed beauty therapist, she also spent several years training in shiatsu, reflexology, aromatherapy massage, colour and sound therapy, lymphatic drainage massage, crystal healing, individual therapy and, most recently, Aurum Manus® therapy with Ricky Welch. Massage has played a constant part in her life for the past 20 years.

Whatever part of the body she is working on — muscles, tendons, joints, connective tissue, lymph glands or skin, and even the less tangible reflex zones and meridians, to Monika the human body is like an open book, in which she is able to 'read' not only physical but also emotional and spiritual disease.

It is from this intimate knowledge and understanding of the body that Monika has

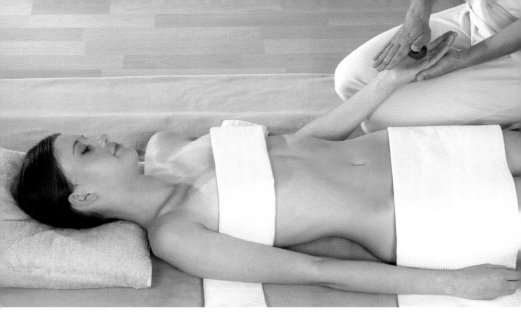

developed her massage methods, and for the last ten years she has also incorporated crystals in her treatments. She explains, 'The interaction between massage strokes and the appropriate crystals enables me to bring about changes in a single massage session that would otherwise only be possible after four or five treatments.' In spite of some initial scepticism on the part of her clients, most are willing to try her methods and are quickly convinced.

Monika's goal in using crystals in massage is to improve the wellbeing of the client, not just in the short term but rather more permanently. She aims for a lasting effect that will help her clients to cope with life's problems and challenges and deal with them in a more relaxed and positive manner.

Such a sense of wellbeing can only be built on a foundation of inner harmony. But what exactly is this 'inner harmony'? We think of something as possessing harmony when its different parts are in balance with each other – therefore, harmony can be created by balancing out any excess or lack. This is why Monika calls her massage system 'Crystal Balance' – it promotes beauty through a sense of wellbeing and harmony created by bringing into balance the different parts of a person's nature and life.

As our state of mind – our mental attitude, approach to life and even mood – is often reflected physically in our bodies, massage enables us to reach the body, mind and spirit all at the same time.

For Monika, it is this holistic approach that forms the basis of 'Crystal Balance'.

It is why her back massage helps you to 'walk tall', a facial massage encourages you to 'show your face' and a leg and foot massage helps you 'get back on your feet'.

Monika deliberately keeps the use of Crystal Balance simple. It is not intended to be a therapy in the medical sense, but rather a treatment programme designed to aid the relaxation and recuperation of the body, working in conjunction with the mind and spirit, encouraging you to 'be yourself'! If we can be who we are, then we are beautiful. It's as simple as that!

I am delighted that Monika Grundmann is now publishing her 'Crystal Balance' and is making it available through seminars and training programmes. Her crystal massage is tried and tested, and easy to learn and perform. Treatments can be carried out as easily at home as in a professional setting by a beauty therapist or as part of a therapeutic treatment. It's not necessary to use all seven steps in a progressive sequence – they can be used individually if

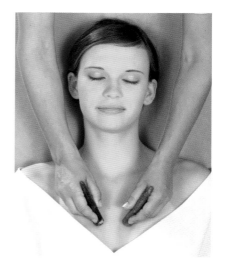

time is short, or you wish to concentrate on one particular aspect, such as interaction with the outside world, experiencing a sense of liberation or simply feeling 'sunshine in your tummy'. But the total body massage is best of all. And what *is* beautiful makes *you* beautiful . . .

Tübingen, Spring 2006
Michael Gienger

9

Crystal Balance

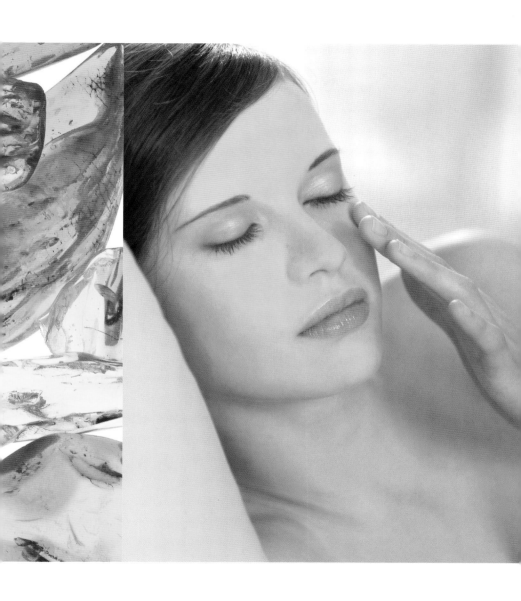

Beauty comes from within. When we are worn out through stress or lack of sleep or trying to deal with life's problems, a quick glance in the mirror can make us cringe – the face we see staring back at us reflects all our troubles. All our efforts to make ourselves look better seem a complete waste of time. In my profession as a beauty therapist, I am often asked to come up with quick-fix solutions to bring out the natural beauty that lies within all of us.

But this cannot be done with cosmetics alone – inner peace and harmony are essential components of beauty. It is with this belief in mind that I have, over the years, developed the system of massage with crystals that I now call Crystal Balance.

The word 'cosmetics' comes from the Greek word *cosmein*, meaning 'ordering and adorning' – which accurately describes the nature of true beauty care. First comes the 'ordering' – creating balance and harmony within ourselves – and then comes the 'adorning', the application of beauty products. If we carry out the 'ordering' process correctly, then the 'adorning' process takes on a secondary, supplementary role rather than being the sole means of beauty care.

'Ordering' allows beauty to shine through our inner wellbeing rather than through any external corrective treatments. In my daily work as a natural beauty therapist and health consultant, I do not set out to heal with crystals in the medicinal sense, but I have found that many people report

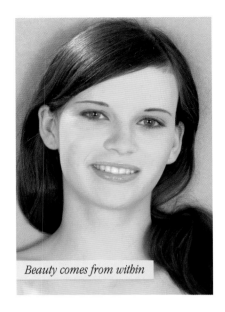

Beauty comes from within

improvements after treatment, such as having fewer migraine attacks or digestive problems, or being able to cope better with stress. So it's no wonder that this 'beauty care' produces better and longer-lasting results.

I see Crystal Balance as a targeted preventive method for maintaining health and beauty. When I am performing a massage, I pick up on the emotions and feelings of the person being massaged and I consciously allow myself to flow totally into what my hands are doing.,

Everything I have learned during my training and years spent practising as a natural-health beauty therapist, even things I thought I had long forgotten, comes together intuitively.

In this way, whatever my instinct tells me is required – colour, sound, aromatic oils, Bach flower remedies – flows into the treatment. This is one of the wonderful things about Crystal Balance – everyone can do it. The way Crystal Balance is used depends on the personality and individual circumstances of the person receiving the massage – the practitioner can then use their knowledge and experience of other therapies to enhance and complement the treatment. This is true for both professional alternative practitioners and those who simply like to share massages at home with a partner.

How can beauty be achieved through touch?

With an average total surface area of almost two square metres, the skin is our largest sensory organ. It contains thousands of nerve endings that respond to stimuli such as pressure and temperature. These nerve endings are particularly concentrated in the more sensitive parts of the body – for example, they are more concentrated on the face and hands than on the back. These sense receptors enable even the faintest and most subtle of sensory impressions to be relayed to the brain at lightning speed. When we are being touched in a pleasurable way, a real cocktail of hormones, including dopamine, oxytocin and endorphins, is produced and poured into the bloodstream. These hormones give us feelings of lightness and happiness, helping to produce an emotional 'high'. According to university studies, the network of nerve endings in our bodies responds particularly well to slow movement; but everything in modern life seems to involve speed. We rush here and there, moving rapidly from one situation to another, bombarded by all kinds of sensory stimulation that initially causes stress and ultimately leads to a dulling and blunting of feeling and perception. In sharp contrast, in Crystal Balance treatment the crystals are passed across the skin with quiet, attentive movements, in circles, by stroking, or with gentle pressure. The treatment reawakens our conscious perception and, even after just a short time, we being to relax. You only have to look at the facial expression of a person receiving massage – they look more open, relaxed and natural, and so much more beautiful!

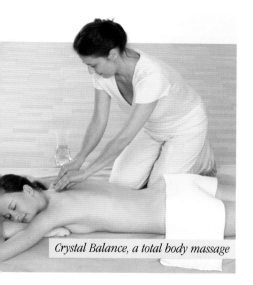

Crystal Balance, a total body massage

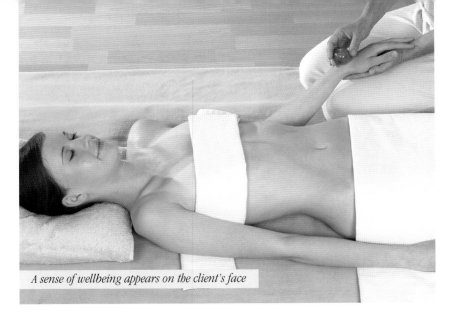

A sense of wellbeing appears on the client's face

There is also a clear connection between a healthy psyche and our immunity to stressful external influences. If we achieve a state of peace and happiness within, we are less likely, for example, to succumb to depression caused by our emotional environment, even if we have inherited a genetic tendency towards depression.

Since it is not a 'healing' treatment, but a beauty care or wellbeing massage, Crystal Balance provides the best opportunities for improving the relationship between people and their emotional environment – without the heavy burden of expectation. It works through touch and helps re-sensitize us to life and the people around us. It helps make life more beautiful for us – and so logically we become more beautiful, too!

I am often asked whether it is possible to do anything to prevent the appearance of wrinkles, and I always give the same answer, explaining that there are 'optimistic wrinkles' and 'pessimistic wrinkles', and that we will do our best to make sure that our clients' wrinkles are only the optimistic kind. I have always thought that those old people whose faces are covered in a network of wrinkles simply radiate life experience, dignity, wisdom and beauty.

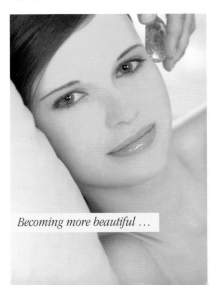

Becoming more beautiful …

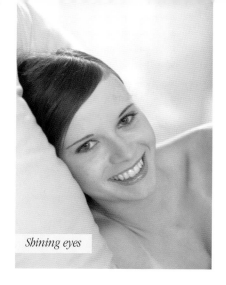

Shining eyes

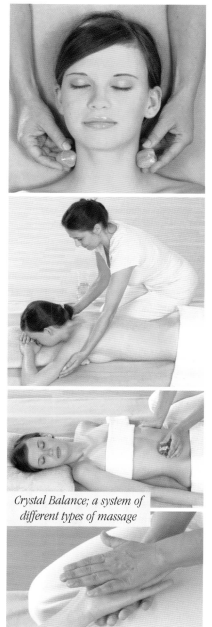

Crystal Balance; a system of different types of massage

It still makes me happy to see how different my clients look after a session of Crystal Balance. Their features look softer, their eyes glow, their entire demeanour changes, their posture is more upright and they walk with more confidence and a definite spring in their step. It is achieving this feeling of inner harmony that is the goal of Crystal Balance. This is what makes us 'beautiful'!

The Crystal Balance method is designed in such a way that it can easily be incorporated into a variety of wellbeing treatments. Over the years I have developed many different steps within the system and each step can be used separately as appropriate, such as for treating the hands, feet, face, back or other specific parts of the body. I invariably carry out a facial cleansing during my beauty care treatments, but the wellbeing part of the treatment is always individually tailored to suit my client. I sense the individual needs of my client and then put together the appropriate treatment session – rather like composing a musical symphony.

How did Crystal Balance originate?

Crystal massage has become an increasingly important element of the range of treatments I offer as a beauty therapist and health consultant. I based the development of Crystal Balance partly on the knowledge derived from my training in crystal healing with Michael Gienger and partly on the tried and tested traditional massage strokes that I have learned over the last 15 years. Experience has shown that the results are even better when, between the applications of crystals or massages with crystals, the client is massaged directly with the hands.

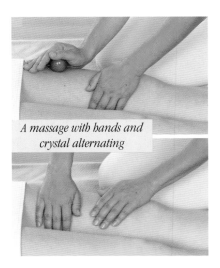

A massage with hands and crystal alternating

This is why I have called this treatment method 'Crystal Balance'.

Not everyone has time for a full Crystal Balance session, which can last up to two hours, so if necessary I choose to leave out certain steps or shorten the treatment as appropriate. But I always complete a full single massage step, so I will treat, for example, both legs for a slightly shorter period of time – but always both legs, never just one! Or I will treat the face only, or the feet, the tummy or the back. It is also extremely important that the massage is carried out harmoniously, calmly and with great care.

I would now like to introduce the seven basic steps of Crystal Balance Total Body Massage, with the accompanying basic movements. Once you have some experience of using these basic steps, you can use your intuition to respond to the individual needs of the person being massaged – we'll call this person your 'massage partner' and refer to 'her', although it is equally suitable for 'him'! – and you can devise your own crystal massage treatments.

During training sessions, my students explore using elements of other alternative treatments during Crystal Massage, such as acupressure, reflexology and meridian treatment, but to explain these in detail here is beyond the scope of this book.

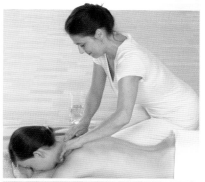

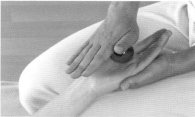

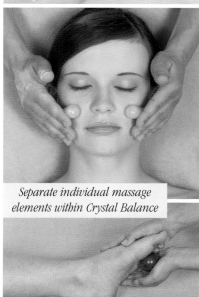

Separate individual massage
elements within Crystal Balance

The Crystal Balance method has been developed from the use of massage and crystals in health and wellbeing. Each of the different sections from the Total Body Massage can be used separately in individual treatments, such as for the back, hands, face or feet. You can also combine it with classic applications – foot care using the foot massage (see page 53) or cosmetic treatment using the facial and upper chest massage (see page 63 and 72).

Do you need massage oils to perform Crystal Balance?

One of the first questions people usually ask at my seminars is whether crystal massage should be carried out with or without oils. The answer is essentially both. There are some situations where the surface tension of the skin should remain unchanged, either for the therapeutic effect (for example, in vital body massage), or for awareness and diagnosis (for example, in reflexology). For more on this, please see Michael Gienger's *Crystal Massage for health and healing* (Earthdancer Books, 2006). However, using a warm, good-quality oil during a Crystal Balance treatment can be extremely beneficial, as it helps the crystals to slide over the skin and also encourages and deepens relaxation of the skin and the body.

I began to use both warm and cool crystals for massaging when I was training with Michael Gienger ten years ago in the use of crystals in holistic beauty care treatments.

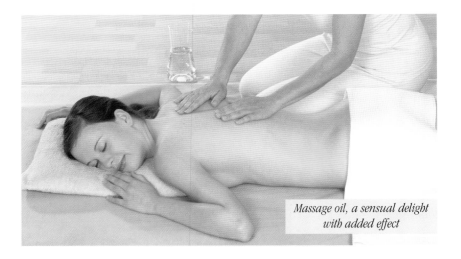

Massage oil, a sensual delight with added effect

When experimenting with creams and oils to ease the movement of the crystals across the skin, I found that plant-based oils turned out to be most suitable. I gradually developed a combination of plant-based oil and certified organic essential oils for use with crystals. My experience in aromatherapy was of great help here – simple trial and error has enabled me to learn which combinations will achieve the best results. For example, I am still impressed by the result that can be achieved by using rose massage oil with Rose Quartz.

When an oil and crystal pairing is particularly effective, my clients experience deep feelings of sensuality, joy and being at one with the world, of really opening up and being receptive to life. At such times the crystal, the oil and the flower essences contained in the oil all seem to come together,

enhancing each other to produce an intense experience.

Preparing mixtures using aromatherapy and essential oils is too wide a field to be covered in this book, but here is a brief insight into what is possible using only crystals and a plant-based oil of your choice.

Combining crystals and oils

Oils that have had crystals bathing in them for a period of time seem to be particularly effective for a Crystal Balance treatment. If a carefully cleansed crystal is placed in a good-quality oil and left to stand in a warm place, the oil will absorb information from the crystal and develop its own effects.

Using both the crystal and the oil in which it has been bathing enhances their potency and results in a very special massage session.

I find the following crystal combinations in massage oils to be particularly effective in Crystal Balance. You can produce these mixtures yourself if you like, but I would recommend that you do this only if you have some background knowledge of aromatherapy. These special crystal oil mixtures, enhanced with different essential oils, can be obtained from specialist suppliers in the UK and US (see appendix p. 106). Choose the appropriate combination by looking at the effect you wish to achieve (such as serenity, security, etc.), or, if you feel more of a connection to the crystals themselves, by looking at the crystals used in the oil-mixtures.

Serenity

Blue Quartz, Dumortierite, Magnesite
Essential oils used: lavender, rosewood, tangerine, roman camomile
This oil promotes deep relaxation; it helps you to unwind and let go, put things into perspective and find inner peace. It is a wonderful oil to use for a massage after a strenuous day. It helps you to see life more positively. It is also very good for stress-related skin problems.

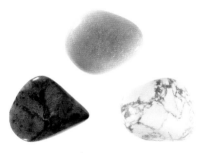

Blue Quartz,
Dumortierite, Magnesite

Security

White Agate, Nephrite, Serpentine
Essential oils used: vanilla, sandalwood, benzoin
This oil helps you to feel secure and protected, and strengthens self-confidence. It helps you to connect with your 'centre', promoting sensitivity and commitment. It brings harmony and inner peace. It also helps you to become more self-aware and creative. A lovely oil also to use for those with restless, quick-tempered natures.

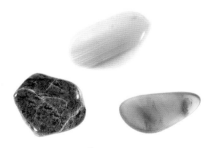

White Agate,
Nephrite, Serpentine

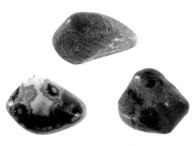

Epidote (Unakite),
Ocean Agate, Zoisite with Ruby

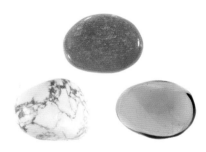

Aventurine,
Magnesite, Smoky Quartz

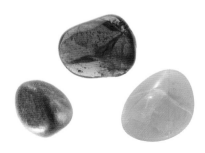

Garnet,
Ruby, Rose Quartz

Regeneration

Epidote (Unakite), Ocean Agate, Zoisite with Ruby
Essential oils used: ravintsara, myrrh, litsea cubeba

Use this oil to restore energy levels and to help you get back on your feet again. It aids mental and physical recovery, enabling you to accomplish more and feel better equipped to cope with problems. It is especially good at times of crisis for those who want to help themselves so that they can enjoy life to the full once again.

Anti-stress

Aventurine, Magnesite, Smoky Quartz
Essential oils used: sweet orange, rose-wood, lavender, ylang ylang

This oil is particularly good for helping you to deal with stress and feel more able to cope with problems. It helps you to face up to things with an inner strength and calm. It is also good for coping with life's daily stresses and strains and helps you to over-come nervousness and anxiety.

Joy of Life

Garnet, Ruby, Rose Quartz
Essential oils used: rose, sandalwood, rose geranium, bergamot

An oil that counteracts sadness and helps you to live life energetically, cheerfully, sensuously and joyfully, with courage and with love.

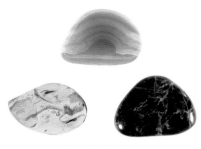

Blue Chalcedony,
Amber, Sodalite

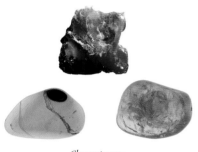

Chrysoprase,
Green Fluorite, Peridot

In the Flow

Blue Chalcedony, Amber, Sodalite
Essential oils used: white fir, geranium,
palmarosa

This oil is particularly good for encouraging energy flow on a physical, emotional and spiritual level. Many problems arise through 'blockages' on these levels. This oil is excellent for toxin removal and also for beauty care.

Fountain of Youth

Chrysoprase, Green Fluorite, Peridot
Essential oils used: juniper berry, sweet
fennel, lemon

Our feeling of wellbeing often depends on the amount of toxins in our bodies. This oil is ideal for detox treatments and should always be part of a detox cure. It helps make the skin more beautiful, and, as with all detox treatments, it not only helps the body to rid itself of toxins but also helps you to release any negative behaviour patterns, so that you feel freer and can become more independent.

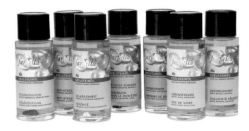

Crystal oils – special compositions
for Crystal Balance made with
the above crystals

The sky really is the limit when it comes to combining crystals and oils – just use your imagination along with a touch of intuition. For example, why not try the oil called 'Happiness', with Garnet, Ruby and Rose Quartz, to treat cold feet; or 'Recovery' at the end of a long, sleepless night. You can obtain crystal oils from specialist cosmetics and crystal suppliers (for suppliers, see Appendix) or you can create your own at home. To produce your own oils, first place a cleansed crystal of your choice (one that has been rubbed vigorously under running water then left to stand on an Amethyst druse for a whole day for energetic charging) in 50ml of good-quality plant oil. Jojoba oil is ideal, as it does not turn rancid too quickly. Then allow the crystal to bathe in the oil for four weeks, in a warm, light place that is as free from environmental stress as possible. After four weeks the oil will have absorbed information from the crystal and can then be used in a treatment.

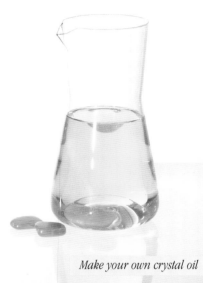

Make your own crystal oil

You can leave the crystal in the dish containing the oil until all the oil has been used up. A list of the various crystals and their properties can be found at the end of the book.

Important: Petroleum-based oils are not suitable for use as base oils, as they do not absorb information particularly well and their consistency reduces the effect of the crystal to some extent. They are not normally good for the skin; they may even block the pores and cause a build-up of toxins. This is why you should always use the very best plant-based oils. I use jojoba oil as the base for my crystal oils. It is a little more expensive, but it has the advantage of almost never going off. It also has almost no scent of its own, which allows the aroma of any essential oils that you add to come out unhindered. If you find that you have used up all your massage base oil, a good-quality olive oil from your kitchen cupboard will also work quite well.

Provided you use a good-quality oil, and not too much of it, you should not need to worry about your client feeling too 'oily' after a massage session. It is surprising just how much oil the skin can absorb.

It is very pleasant and relaxing to have the hair stroked back from the face during a massage. If you intend to do this, do ensure you advise your client beforehand, so that they are prepared to have their hair touched (and their hairstyle possibly disturbed a little!). In the context of the treatment session and the benefits that your client will feel, most will be happy for you to do this.

> A Crystal Balance treatment is carried out with oil that has been warmed. You will need to use a good-quality plant-based oil (such as jojoba, sesame or almond), a combination oil that you have made yourself, or a ready-made crystal oil that you have bought.

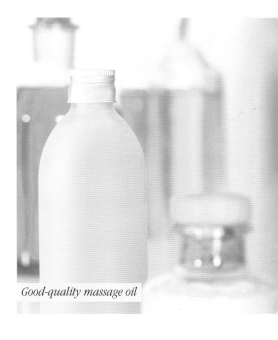
Good-quality massage oil

Warm and cool crystals

The effects of the Crystal Balance treatment are intensified when the oils and crystals are warmed. Warmth enhances the relaxation process, and your client will be more receptive to the effects of the crystals. In some massages, using cool crystals alongside warm ones can have a very useful and stimulating effect.

However, I only use only warmed crystals to perform Crystal Balance, or crystals that are at room temperature, but never cold ones. Crystals that have been kept at room temperature will in any case feel cool to the client. I use cool crystals in specific areas only and usually only for a brief period, for example, around the eyes at the end of a facial treatment. They feel extremely refreshing and, when used at the end of a massage, help wake the client up again in a gentle and pleasant way. They also encourage good circulation and oxygen supply to the tissues.

What is the best method of warming the crystals?

I have tried lots of different methods, but have recently decided that warming them in a bath of oil over a small burner is still the best way, as using electrical appliances always runs the risk of electromagnetic pollution. The Crystal Balance work trolley was developed during training sessions and is an extremely useful working tool. Tea lights can be placed in containers and the amount of heat they give out can be controlled by adjusting their height individually. The trolley can be pushed around the treatment table quite easily with one hand while you are massaging the client with the other. This allows you to remain in contact with the client's body throughout, which is important, as explained previously. The crystals, singing bowls and other treatment equipment needed, fit neatly into the spaces designed specifically for them (sources are listed at the end of the book).

For a complete Crystal Balance session you need:

- Around 30ml of warm oil per dish.
- Two warmed rod-shaped crystals for the feet (just the blunt ends can be placed in oil beforehand) and another two crystal rods for the face.
- Two warmed palmstone crystals.
- One or two crystal spheres.
- A smooth crystal (for example, rock crystal slices or tumbled crystals) or spherical crystal at room temperature, for stimulation.
- A dish for the crystal rods to be used for the feet and for the palmstone crystals.
- A second dish for the crystal rods for the face and for the sphere(s).
- Crystal Balance work trolley (for sources see appendix p. 106)

To begin with, while your collection of crystals and oils is still fairly small, you can use fewer crystals.

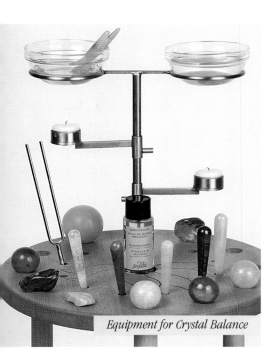

Equipment for Crystal Balance

Creating the right atmosphere

The easiest way to carry out a crystal massage treatment is to have your massage partner lying on a table that is accessible from all sides. You can also carry out a massage on the floor, providing you find this comfortable. As with all kinds of massage, warmth, calmness and a comfortable position for your massage partner are important. Make sure that you have everything you need easily to hand before you actually start the session.

One of the most important rules is, 'Always maintain contact with your partner during the massage session'. By this I mean that one hand should always be touching the body, even if you are fetching an item with your other hand. You will therefore need to have the work trolley positioned fairly close to your massage partner so that you can easily access your equipment. Make sure also that there are enough towels or sheets within reach to cover up the areas of the body that are not being treated. Pleasant surroundings and the right atmosphere will

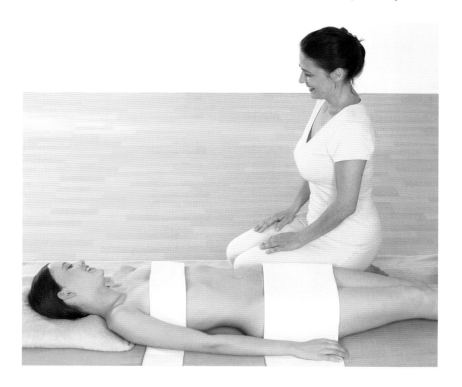

Getting the right atmosphere:
- The room temperature should be as comfortably warm as possible.
- The lighting should be soft.
- No mobile phones or telephones are allowed!
- No jewellery or watches, and preferably no spectacles, either for you or your massage partner.
- A comfortable massage table or a well-padded but firm massage surface.
- Sufficient towels or sheets to cover your massage partner.
- Warmed oils and crystals, ready for the massage, **but check that the temperature is no more than hand-hot (35°C).**
- Soothing background music, providing your massage partner likes this.

Keep within easy reach during the massage:
- The prepared work trolley.
- Crystals warmed in oil.
- Cool crystals (at room temperature).

After the massage:
- Make sure there is plenty of water available. (I have noticed that my clients frequently need to drink water after – and sometimes during the massage – and you may wish to drink water too.)

greatly increase the success of the massage. But the most important requirement for a successful treatment is your own attentiveness and desire to achieve the best outcome – to help your massage partner achieve what they want from the treatment.

During a training session in 'Individual Therapy' with Rainer Strebel, I learned another valuable lesson. If you are able to connect with your higher self and be in tune with the needs of your client, provided you work carefully and with concentration you will find that the appropriate moves come to you naturally and instinctively. I mention this by way of encouragement to any beginner who may be feeling a little daunted by the vast array of crystals and oils available, and all the techniques that have to be learned.

Choosing crystals

If you are using Crystal Balance for the first time, I recommend that you only use one type of crystal initially with each massage, so that you can note the different effects each crystal has. Later, when you have more experience, you will gain in confidence and be able to enjoy using a combination of crystals to suit each individual. You can also 'dowse' for the appropriate crystal using kinesiology (muscle-testing), a pulse diagnostic or a one-handed dowsing device. I like to use a one-handed dowsing rod, as my client can be quite relaxed throughout and does not have to do anything while I am testing. That is why I teach this method of dowsing in my training sessions – and there is usually a huge sigh of relief from people attending the course, who until then have been finding the vast array of available crystals totally confusing.

You should normally work with pairs of crystal rods, palmstones or spheres. I like to recommend Rose Quartz or Serpentine for those attempting crystal massage for the first time, as both have a pleasant, gentle effect.

When you have more experience, choosing crystals that suit the needs of your client will help make your treatments more successful. Before you begin the massage, take the time to talk to your client so that you can gauge their wishes and needs. The sec-

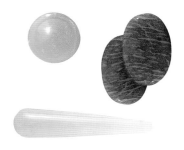

Crystal sphere, rod and palmstones

tion that follows suggests which are the best crystals to use for each purpose. For ease of reference, they are not shown here as rods, palmstones and spheres, but as tumbled crystals. But you can choose the crystal that is the most suitable and pleasant for the massage you are going to perform.

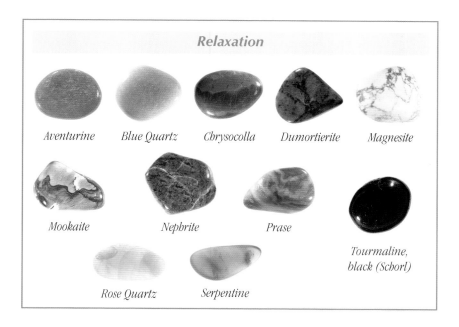

Relaxation

Aventurine   *Blue Quartz*   *Chrysocolla*   *Dumortierite*   *Magnesite*

Mookaite   *Nephrite*   *Prase*

Tourmaline, black (Schorl)

Rose Quartz   *Serpentine*

Releasing stress and tension

Amethyst

Fluorite

Magnesite

Tourmaline, black (Schorl)

Moss Agate

Obsidian

Smoky Quartz

Achieving balance

Agate

Amazonite

Amber

Chrysocolla

Mookaite

Moss Agate

Nephrite

Petrified Wood

Prase

Serpentine

Regeneration

Calcite

Chrysocolla

Epidote (Unakite)

Moss Agate

Ocean Agate (Ocean Jasper)

Tiger Iron

Tourmaline, green

Zoisite with Ruby

Increasing energy levels

Halite

Hematite

Jasper, red

Obsidian

Rock Crystal

Tourmaline, black (Schorl)

Tourmaline, green

Tourmalinated Quartz

Staying calm

Amazonite

Aventurine

Blue Quartz

Chrysocolla

Dumortierite

Magnesite

Moss Agate

Prase

Serpentine

Sodalite

Protection and boundaries

Agate

Amber

Aventurine

Halite

Heliotrope

Obsidian

Serpentine

*Tourmaline,
black (Schorl)*

Lifting depression

Amber

Calcite, orange

Citrine

Sunstone

Detoxing and purifying

Amazonite

Amber

Aventurine

Chalcedony, blue

Chrysocolla

Chrysoprase

Fluorite

Halite

Moss Agate   *Nephrite*   *Ocean Agate (Ocean Jasper)*   *Tourmaline, green*

Stimulating lymphatic flow

Amber   *Aquamarine*   *Chalcedony, blue*   *Chrysoprase*   *Heliotrope*

Magnesite   *Moss Agate*   *Ocean Agate (Ocean Jasper)*   *Sodalite*

Improving circulation

Hematite   *Jasper, red*   *Mookaite*   *Obsidian*

Rhodonite   *Rose Quartz*   *Tiger Iron*

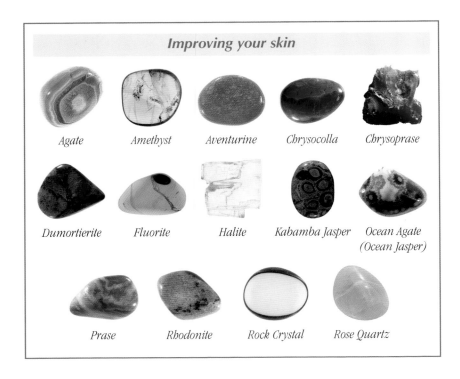

Improving your skin

| Agate | Amethyst | Aventurine | Chrysocolla | Chrysoprase |

| Dumortierite | Fluorite | Halite | Kabamba Jasper | Ocean Agate (Ocean Jasper) |

| Prase | Rhodonite | Rock Crystal | Rose Quartz |

I would like to point out here that the notorious problem of cellulite is really just one of the body's ways of safely storing waste substances (toxins) in the subcutaneous layers of the tissue until they are eliminated by the body's natural detoxification process. The problem is that we allow ourselves far too little time for the body to rest and recuperate these days – even while we are slumping on the sofa watching an action film, our bodies are in a state of tension, which is not conducive to the detoxification process. Our fatty tissue thus becomes a regular 'waste bin'; this is why new mothers who are still breastfeeding should never go on a diet, as the dissolving of fat from the tissues will also dissolve out the toxins, which will then pass into the mother's milk. Women, and even men, are beginning to discover the first signs of cellulite at an increasingly younger age, due to the ever-growing levels of stress in society, eating the wrong kinds of food and lack of exercise.

The important thing to bear in mind when detoxing and purifying the body's systems is that you need not only to eliminate the waste substances from the tissues, but also to encourage the body to function efficiently on a daily basis so that toxins do not build up again.

Further ideas on all the above treatments can be found in the descriptions of crystals at the end of this book. Crystals that are not available as rods, palmstones or spheres (for example, Amber, for use in the wonderful amber-oil massage) can instead be used in the form of tumbled crystals or in other shapes, as long as there are no sharp edges and they are pleasantly smooth to the touch.

It takes at least ten minutes for the crystals to reach the right temperature, so place your chosen crystals in the warm oil in good time before the massage session is to start.

Exercises

The following three exercises will act as a preparation for your first massage, helping you to become familiar with the different shapes and the effects of the crystals. These exercises can be repeated occasionally to help improve and fine-tune your perception and dexterity.

Exercise 1

With your eyes closed, first massage your own face with a finger, then with a crystal rod. Look upon the rod as an extension of your finger, as if the rod actually contains nerve endings too. You will find that your consciousness is extended into the tip of the rod.

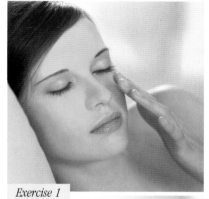

Exercise 1

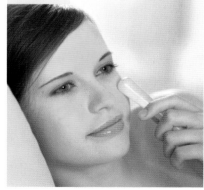

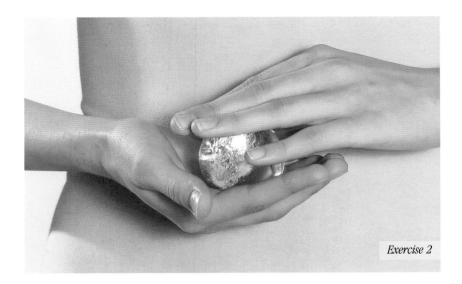

Exercise 2

Roll a crystal sphere slowly in the palms of your hands and note what you are sensing and feeling. Immediately afterwards, select a sphere from another type of crystal and repeat the movement. Do you notice the difference?

Exercise 3

Using two palmstone crystals, massage your own thighs in synchronized circular movements. Try holding the crystals in different ways and work out how they feel best. Also vary the pressure and the speed and note how the massage movements feel to you.

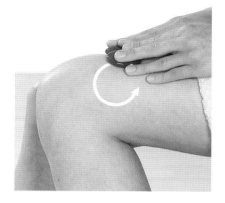

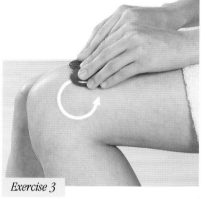

Exercise 3

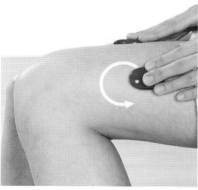

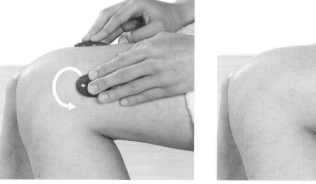

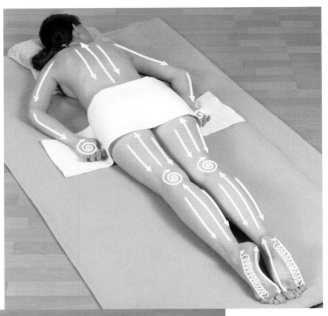

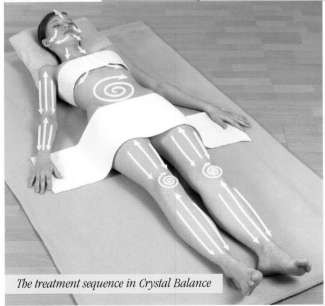

The treatment sequence in Crystal Balance

Crystal Balance – the treatment sequence

The treatment always begins and ends with the feet. Even if I am only carrying out a balancing treatment on the face, I briefly massage the feet too. This is to make an initial contact with my client, and then to say 'goodbye', as it were, after completing the session.

When performing a total body massage, I begin with the client lying in a prone position so that I can massage the legs and back first and then the front of the body, beginning again with the feet, then moving to the hands and arms, the face, the top of the chest, the stomach and finally the legs again. The natural flow of energy runs up the front of the body from the feet to the head and then from the head down the back to the feet again. Trying to massage in the direction of this flow is difficult as the released energy is unable to flow freely if the 'exit' is blocked, so I have found that I can obtain better results by first 'opening up' the back and then working on the front of the body. Therefore I usually massage the back of the body using stroking movements towards the feet. This 'stroking out' movement is an important part of the massage. Whenever I feel the massage is becoming difficult, I see it as a signal that the backed-up energy has to be made to flow again through these 'stroking out' movements.

You will need the following crystals for the Crystal Balance session:

Two crystal rods.
Two palmstone crystals.
Two crystal spheres.
(All the crystals should be of the same type.)

Important: Always check beforehand that the crystals are the right temperature and not too hot – the best way is with the elbow. Remember that the hands and feet can generally withstand more heat than the more sensitive skin of the face.

Crystal Balance –
the techniques

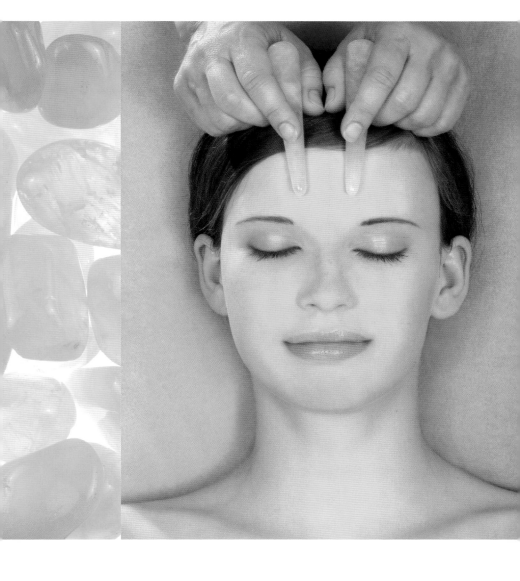

Preparation

Begin the Crystal Balance session with a footbath, gradually increasing in temperature from 35 to 45°C and lasting 15 to 20 minutes. The footbath balances out the emphasis on the head and helps the client to remain grounded. In addition, it promotes relaxation of the whole body, so that the client finds it easier to switch off from everyday matters and tune into the treatment. I use this time to chat to my client over a cup of tea and establish what they would like to gain from the treatment. It often helps to be able to 'read between the lines' when deciding which crystals to use and choosing the right emphasis for the subsequent massage session.

> The Crystal Balance massage begins with a footbath (temperature increasing from 35 to 45°C) which lasts 15 to 20 minutes.
>
> Chat with the client beforehand to help you decide what the emphasis of the massage should be and what type(s) of crystals to use.
>
> Warm the crystals in good time before the session.
>
> Offer the client a drink, and remember to drink yourself too.

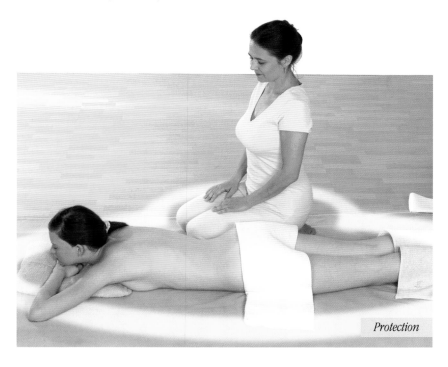

Protection

Protection

Before you begin the massage, create a protective boundary between you and your massage partner. My usual method is to visualize a horizontal figure eight around myself and my client, with me inside one of the loops of the eight and my client in the other. This means we are connected, but without mingling our energies. I also like to start and end my crystal massage sessions using sound created either by a special aluminium tuning fork or by a Tibetan singing bowl, which I move about above my client. The client's aura determines the tuning – with experience, you will be able to use any changes in tone to identify which areas of the body have a 'denseness' that needs addressing, and also get a sense of the emphasis that is required during the treatment. Use the tuning fork or singing bowl again at the end of the session to 'tone out' any energetic 'leftovers'. You will notice that the tone now sounds quite different.

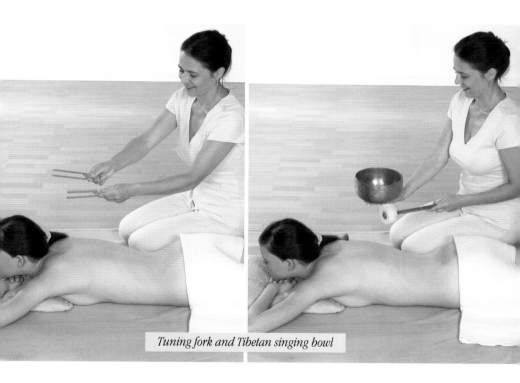

Tuning fork and Tibetan singing bowl

Take the weight off her shoulders

Use two palmstone crystals for the first part of the massage session. You can change the type of crystal you use to suit the different stages of the treatment (feet, legs, back, shoulders, neck).

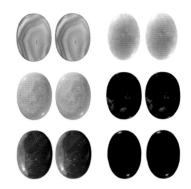

While your massage partner is lying on her tummy, pour some oil on both legs. Spread it over her legs with flowing movements that carry on beyond the soles of the feet, as if you were extending a line into infinity. Then begin the massage using warmed crystals (unless your massage partner has varicose veins, in which case use crystals at room temperature). Cover the parts of the body that are not being treated with a towel or sheet to keep your partner warm.

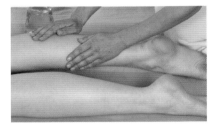

Make sure the crystals are at the right temperature, then gently place one on the sole of the left foot. Then begin, first with light then with firmer pressure, to massage the sole of the foot with circular movements. Apply a little more pressure to the heels and the balls of the foot.

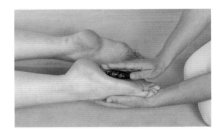

Then massage the heel area with gentle pressure on both sides upwards and downwards. Experiment a little with the way you hold the crystal until it feels comfortably 'round' in your hand.

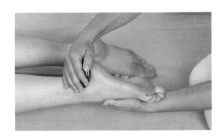

Now draw the crystal a few times from right to left across the heel and back.

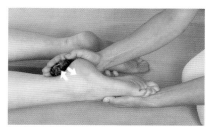

Next, beginning with the Achilles tendon, stroke alternately from right to left, past the ankle bone to the top of the instep and to the tips of the toes. Lift the foot slightly for this.

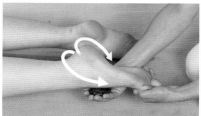

Repeat the movement on the other foot and then lay the crystal back in the dish of oil, remembering to stay connected to your partner with one hand.

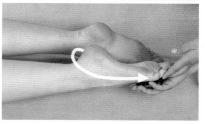

Move the other warmed crystal from the heel over the calf to the back of the knee (take care as this area is sensitive to heat) and alternately down the sides to either the big toe or little toe and beyond.

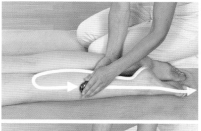

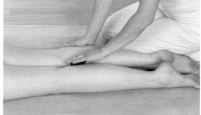

Now take both palmstone crystals and begin massaging to the right and left of the Achilles tendon. Move the crystals up to the buttock, with very little pressure, and then, with a little more pressure, back along the right and left sides of the leg. Repeat this movement several times.

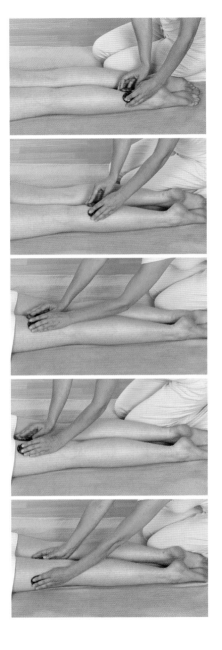

Now, starting at the buttock, stroke the crystals down the middle of the thigh, down along the calf and, with a bit of momentum, across the heel and the soles of the feet down to the toes, just as if you were stroking out everything that is not required.

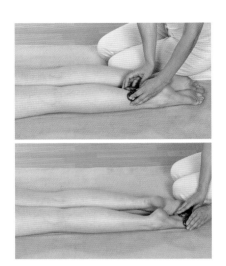

Repeat this up and down massage several times until the leg feels really relaxed. When you reach the foot again, change to the right leg with a fluid motion. When doing this, make contact with your right hand on the right leg, while still maintaining contact for a moment with your left hand on the left foot. Then proceed to massage the right leg in the same way.

After massaging the right leg, briefly lay the crystals back in the warm oil (one hand should always remain in contact with your partner) and take up more oil. Spread this over your partner's back with broad, sweeping movements.

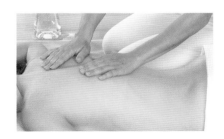

Lay one palmstone crystal gently on the sacral area and then begin to massage with small, then increasingly larger figure-of-eight movements across the entire area of the lower back. The 'knot-point' of the figure-eight shape should always be the spine. *Never exert any kind of pressure when passing over the spine.*

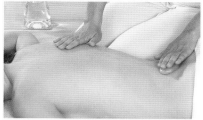

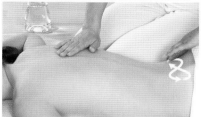

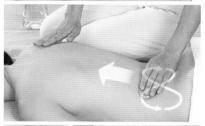

Then continue with the figure-eight movements across the entire back right up to the shoulders. *Again, pay attention never to exert any kind of pressure when passing across the spine.*

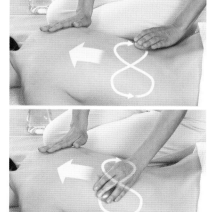

Then stroke the neck, beginning to the right and left of the spine, alternating around twice on each side and moving down towards the buttocks without exerting any pressure on the spine.

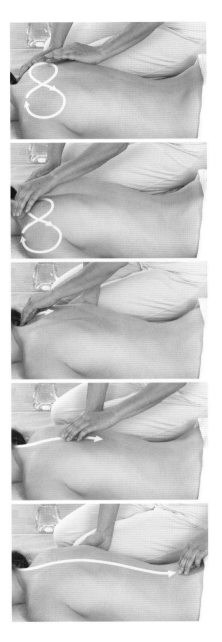

After that, pummel and knead the entire back using two crystals, while once again ensuring that you never ever work directly on the spine. The pummelling motion of both hands should run together, rather like kneading dough. If you sense tension, gentle pressure or patting with the crystal will often be helpful. Be sure to change sides without taking your hands away from your partner's body.

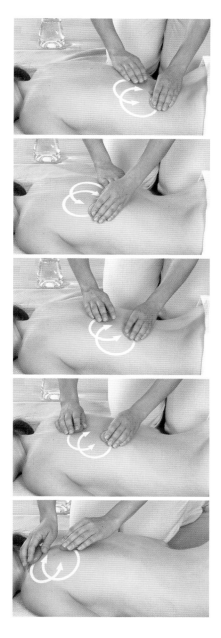

Next, carefully work on the muscles of the shoulders including the shoulder joint, which should be worked around with repeated figure-of-eight movements. Gently massage the edge of the shoulder blade from the centre outward.

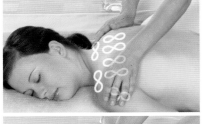

Now move along the neck with a lightly applied upward movement from the sixth neck vertebra to the right and left of the spine up to the hairline. Remain there for a few seconds. Allow the crystal to glide back and repeat this procedure about three times. Afterwards, massage this area gently and carefully with your hands.

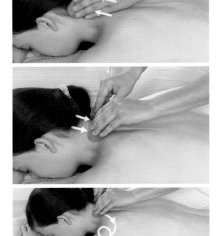

Finally, massage the neck and shoulders on both sides, first progressing in slower circular motions, then in more rapid movements outward along the arms. Always move the crystal back gently to the neck.

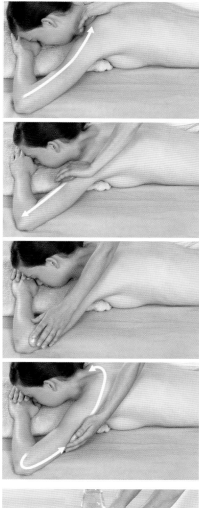

Continue with the stroking movements down the back. Begin on the right and left of the spine with gentle pulling movements right down to the buttocks. Repeat this stroking out movement at least three times.

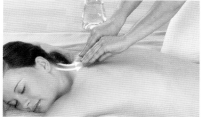

Many people will feel a great sense of liberation if you also continue the movement over the buttocks, down the backs of the thighs to the soles of the feet and beyond.

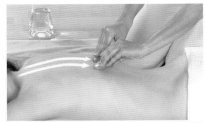

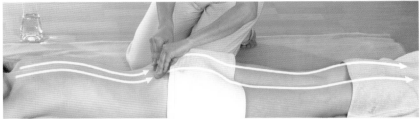

With this back massage alone it is possible to balance the entire body. Along the back are so-called 'Head's zones' (named after their discoverer, Henry Head, 1893). These are reflex zones connected via a direct nerve channel in the spinal marrow with all the internal organs. Crystal massage along the back will stimulate and balance out these zones.

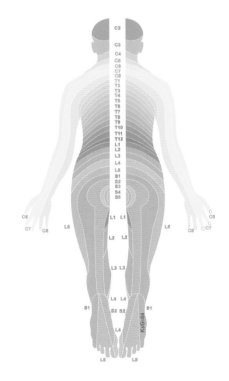

A grounding foot massage

We have a tendency to neglect our feet, but they carry us through our lives and therefore merit particular attention during the Crystal Balance session. In addition, most of the meridians – those energy channels that run through our bodies – end at the toes, while the entire body is reflected in the feet.

For this stage of the massage session your massage partner should be turned on her back and wrapped up warmly. Please make sure that her shoulders are well covered. You should now make sure that one hand is working while the other hand supports the foot. For this stage of the session, you use the crystal rods.

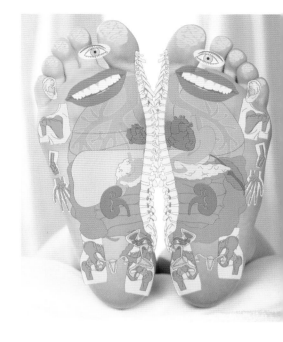

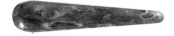

Oil the feet well with a good-quality warmed oil to begin with. Then massage the ankle on both sides of the foot in gentle circular movements using the blunt end of the rod, followed by loop-like movements around the ankle bones.

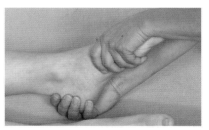

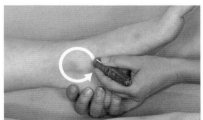

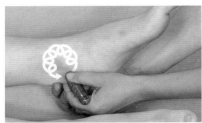

Then use stroking movements with a light drawing action from the toes to the ankle joint (this supports the flow of lymph in the foot and clears blockages).

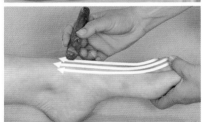

Afterwards, massage the inside of the foot from the toes to the heel with tiny circular movements, without pressure, using the blunt end of the rod. In reflexology terms this corresponds to the spine.

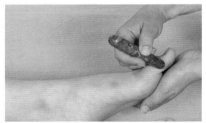

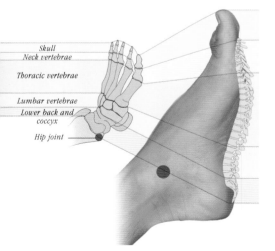

Skull
Neck vertebrae

Thoracic vertebrae

Lumbar vertebrae
Lower back and coccyx

Hip joint

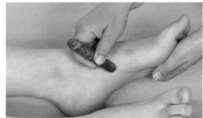

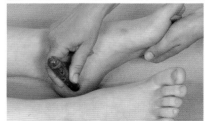

Then, moving in a flowing action from the heel to the ankle joint, slowly stroke (about ten times) the entire upper part of the foot from the ankle joint to the tips of the toes.

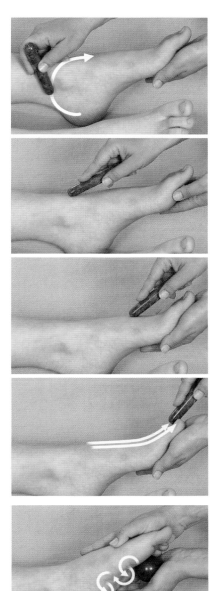

Then massage the sole of the foot from the balls of the toes towards the heel. For this part it is good to work with a warmed crystal sphere. The general rule is that the thicker the skin, the more pressure you can exert.

Of special benefit is the massage along the heel, which corresponds to the pelvic area. The movements should flow together, whether they are circular, spiral or a figure-of-eight shape.

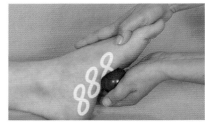

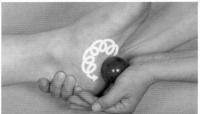

Before changing back from the sphere to the rod, press the sphere gently into the heel. You can support this grip by pressing to the rhythm of your breathing. Allow the sphere to sink in three times.

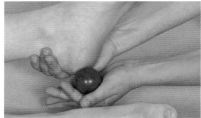

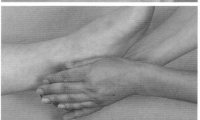

Afterwards, gently massage the inner edge of the foot at pressure points spaced about 1cm apart from the big toe to the heel. With this action, you are working on the reflexology zones of the spine again.

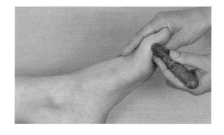

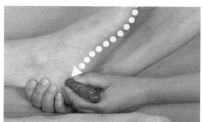

At the end, the foot should be massaged and stroked again, by hand, gently and slowly. Finally, gently pull the individual toes.

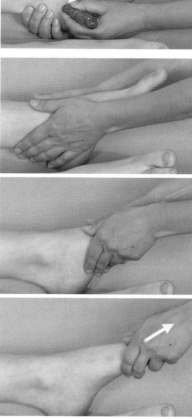

Now wrap the left foot in a warm towel and proceed with massaging the right foot in the same way.

Get to know each other better

We are able to take up and release large amounts of energy through our hands. They are hugely, and intimately, involved with our contact with our environment. In addition, both the hands and feet possess reflex zones and meridian channels. During massage it is noticeable that the second hand relaxes far sooner than the first, as it is reflexively learning from the experience of the first one. Nevertheless, the massage for the second arm should last just as long as for the first. It is precisely at the wrists, elbows and shoulders that the flow of energy is often blocked. Therefore massage these areas particularly thoroughly – but gently – even around the joints. During this part of the massage you will be using a crystal sphere with a diameter of about 3-4cm.

To begin with, place a little massage oil in your massage partner's left hand and on the left arm and gently massage it in.

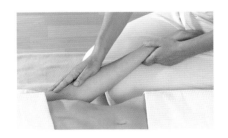

Then take a crystal sphere and massage, initially gently, then a little more firmly, the palms of the hands, including the undersides of the fingers.

With one hand, roll the sphere in small circular movements, while your other hand firmly supports your partner's hand. Move the sphere in such a way that you are constantly circling around a different invisible centre. Observe your partner while you are doing this and vary the pressure applied.

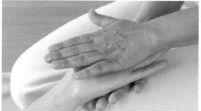

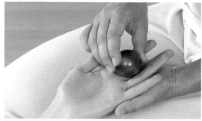

Beginning at the wrist, stroke the individual fingers right down to the fingertips and even beyond a little, as if you were simply drawing out the tension.

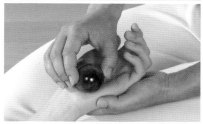

Now draw the sphere to the wrist and gently make figure-of-eight movements across the two little mounds which are visible below the folds of the wrist. This action is called 'sun and moon'.

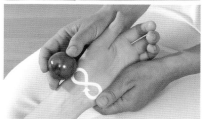

Turn the hand over and draw the sphere from the wrist along the individual fingers and beyond (just as before on the palm of the hand).

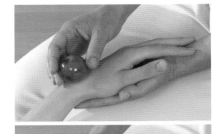

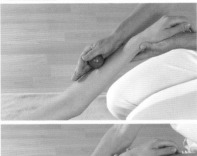

Then begin to stroke along the lower arm using the sphere. Initially, this should be towards the elbow, around it and back. When you have practised this a bit, you can use the sphere alternately in your right and then left hand.

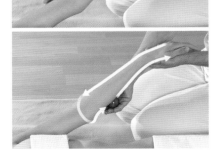

Repeat the same stroking movements on the upper arm. Pay special attention to the shoulder joint; keep on circling around it.

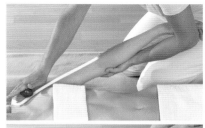

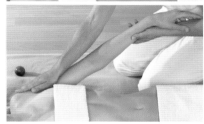

Following on from this, make long stroking movements with your hand along the entire length of the arm. Begin at the shoulders and move down towards the hands.

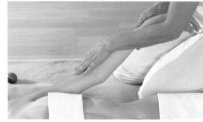

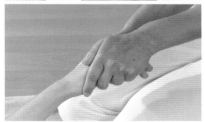

Next, knead the backs of the hands then the palms of the hands again with movements that open outwards.

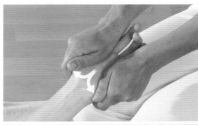

To finish, carefully pull each of the fingers.

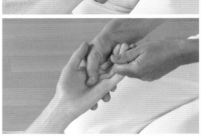

Wrap the left arm in a warm towel and massage the right arm in the same way. Please pay attention here to make sure the transfer from one arm to the other is carried out fluidly.

Reveal the true beauty

By now your massage partner should be lying there in a pretty relaxed state. If this is not the case, check if something is not right with her. I have often noticed that at this point in the treatment the client may feel the need to go to the toilet, but is embarrassed to tell me so. In order to avoid this situation, I always tell her at the beginning of the treatment, when I am offering tea or water, that it is quite normal and a good sign that the body is beginning to get 'into the flow' during the treatment.

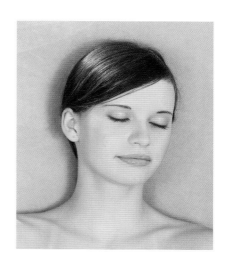

Even in the summer I usually have a *light* woollen blanket ready for covering up on top of the sheet, because, during these intense treatments, the energy of the client is very much 'directed inward' and she will easily feel chilly. If anyone answers your question as to whether they are warm enough with just 'it's OK', then they are probably too cold. Then I will always say, 'OK is not enough', and they are usually quite happy to be covered up.

Less pressure is applied when working on the facial area, especially at the temples. There we will be working with two crystal rods or with two tumbled crystals, used in tandem, which is to encourage bringing the two halves of the brain into balance and is usually perceived as very relaxing. Please make sure that the crystals are not too hot when using them for the facial massage!

Place a little warmed oil on the face, neck and top of the chest. Distribute the oil with gentle, circular movements.

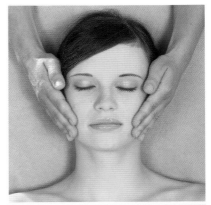

Using tumbled Blue Chalcedony crystals, begin massaging the neck with very delicate, stationary circles from the ear lobes to the hollow of the collarbone, working downwards about a finger's width at a time. Avoid the area around the thyroid cartilage (Adam's apple). Repeat this movement three times. Together, this massage technique and the effect of the Blue Chalcedony will stimulate the lymph flow and prepare your partner in an optimal fashion for the facial massage.

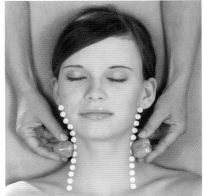

Now place the blunt ends of the crystal rods at the bridge of the nose and gently draw them up across the head as far as possible. Then stroke down behind the ears and on down to the shoulders. Follow this with the same movement from the centre of the eyebrows and finally start from the outer edges of the eyebrows.

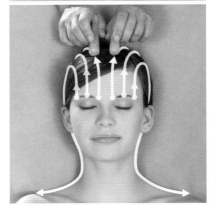

Then stroke the forehead, starting from the centre, towards the temples and beyond. Start on the eyebrows with the first stroking movements and end at the hairline (or wherever it would be...). Work your way from the eyebrows, moving upwards by a finger-width at a time. The gentle stroking movements across the forehead should extend down almost to the table or surface on which your massage partner is lying.

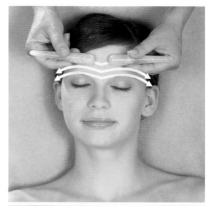

Then hold the rods by the blunt end so that they are lying flat on the forehead. Using rotating alternating movements, massage the entire width of the forehead through to the hairline.

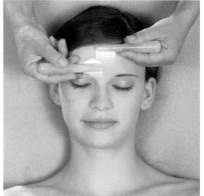

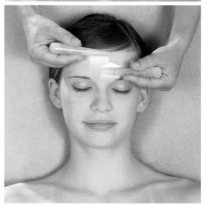

Next, for a moment, fix on the acupressure point between the inner corner of the eye and the inner edge of the eyebrows. This point lies on the bladder meridian and also helps promote a deeper level of relaxation.

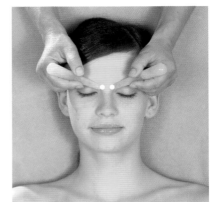

Now draw the rod (with slight pressure in the direction of the forehead) several times across the eyebrows towards the temples and allow the movement to peter out behind the ear. *Attention: No pressure should be applied to the temples.*

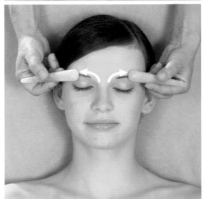

Then place the rods directly on the temples and move them in an extremely delicate spiral movement towards you. This action helps with the releasing of pressure from the head area.

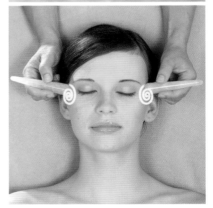

Now, starting at the bridge of the nose, massage the entire area of the cheeks in small, figure-of-eight movements down to the chin.

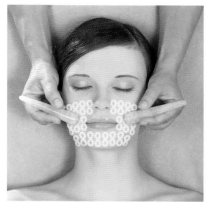

Please pay special attention to the muscles of the jaw in front of and below the ear. Even tight circles will encourage the release of much tension here.

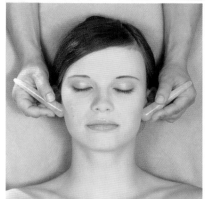

After that, roll the rods from the top downward across the cheeks several times.

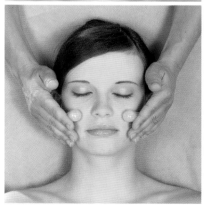

Now massage the lower jaw in small circular movements, beginning from the centre of the chin to the jaw joint.

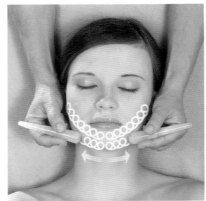

Afterwards, massage the upper jaw with small circular movements from under the nose and under the cheekbones towards the jaw joint.

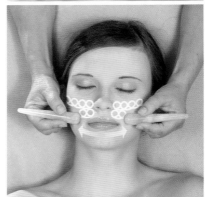

The following action is called 'Yin-Yang Balance'. Place the rod tip gently on the pressure point above the upper lip in the dimple and the other rod tip horizontally below the lower lip. Remain in this position for about 10 seconds and then very gently change the rods, so that the rod that was initially at the top is now at the bottom and vice versa.

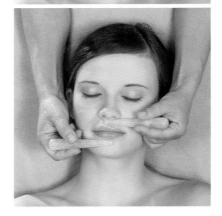

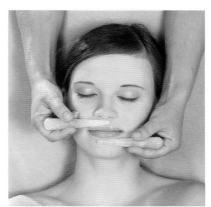

Finally – as at the beginning – set the lymph flow of the neck in motion once again with the tumbled Chalcedony crystals.

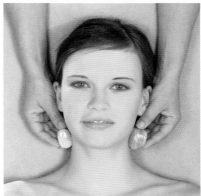

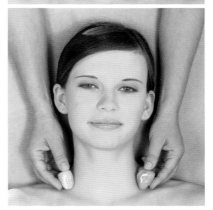

At the end, lay two flat Rock Crystal slices on the eyes for about 30 seconds, or gently stroke the area around the eyes with the cool crystal.

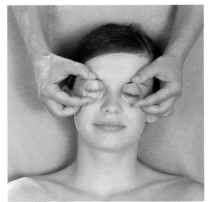

After that, stroke the entire face once more in a fan-like movement with the hands.

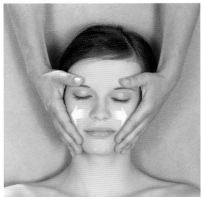

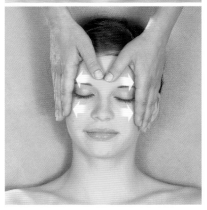

Tip: In cases of severe tension in the muscles of the jaw, placing a piece of Smoky Quartz, which is as flat as possible, on the area in front of the ear and then placing a tuning fork at a level of 240Hz on the crystal has proven to be very beneficial.

After placing the tuning fork in this position two or three times, the vibrating effect will cause the surrounding tissue to relax. Repeat this procedure on the other side. The result with one of my clients was amazing. She looked quite different and even noticed this herself. She had a much softer facial expression and then told me that, during the treatment with the tuning fork, much of what had been causing her stress had simply 'flown away' on the sound.

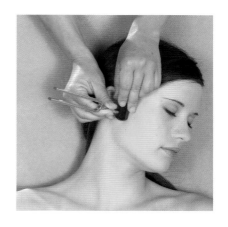

Rose Quartz has proven very effective for the facial treatment. With Rose Quartz the skin actually looks 'rosier', with improved blood circulation, and is softer and more relaxed. For the massage I use 'Joie de Vivre' oil with the vibrational energy of Rose Quartz and also pure rose oil (or rose massage oil). I refer to particularly extended Crystal Balance facial massage sessions with Rose Quartz and rose oil as 'Rose Quartz harmony'.

Feel free!

Bad posture and internal tension cause the muscles between our ribs – the muscles that essentially influence our breathing – to be tense most of the time. During my treatments, especially with the massage of the upper chest area, I often find that my clients suddenly breathe in deeply, as if they have just been liberated from a tight band around their chest. Their breathing becomes freer and a deep sense of wellbeing floods in. I usually massage the upper chest with well-warmed crystal rods or crystal spheres and warm oil. The warmth causes the muscles to relax even more easily.

Initially, massage the entire upper chest from the centre of the sternum upwards and outwards to the shoulders, alternating in circles and stroking, first by hand, then with the rods.

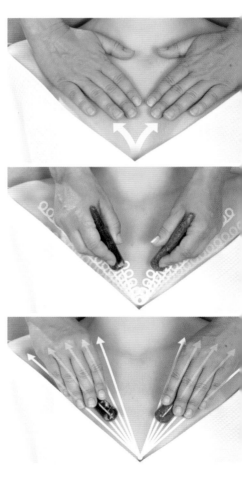

Then try to find the areas between the ribs and stimulate them with rhythmic, point-like movements towards the outside. The pressure points end under the collarbone.

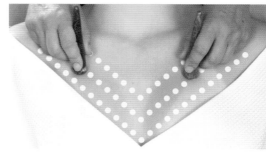

At the end, stroke once again with the hands as if you were trying to pull the breast cage apart, always moving along the course of the ribs from the sternum towards the shoulders.

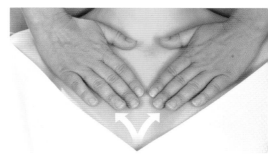

Please ensure, when massaging, to work between the ribs (particularly pleasant) and not on the ribs (particularly unpleasant)! Mookaite and Moss Agate have proven to be especially beneficial for this massage.

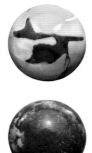

Warm sun in your tummy

Do you know that feeling of warm sun shining in your tummy and feeling just so good and relaxed inside? The solar plexus has a central role to play in expressing our joie de vivre. Unfortunately, we pay far too little attention to the 'tummy', apart from moaning about rolls of fat. But the fact that the tummy is of great significance is expressed in using such expressions as 'good feelings', or having 'a good feeling inside'. So, let our tummies have a share of what they deserve – warmth and stroking of the best kind!

In most cases I use Mookaite spheres for the tummy massage. However, particularly good alternatives, especially for women, are massage with Malachite (in cases of cramp and tension in the lower tummy area and for encouraging sensuality) or Moonstone (for that gut feeling and during menstruation), as well as Emerald (for strengthening the immune system, for harmonizing the gut and for general regeneration).

At the beginning of the massage, distribute well-warmed oil in circular stroking movements across the tummy (clockwise).

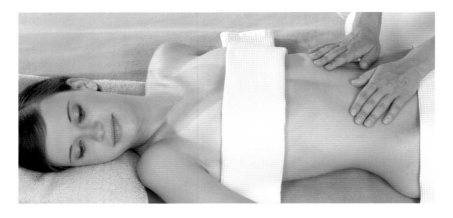

Then lay the warmed sphere on the navel for a few seconds. Afterwards, gently move the sphere about three times clockwise across the tummy, taking into consideration the course of the intestine.

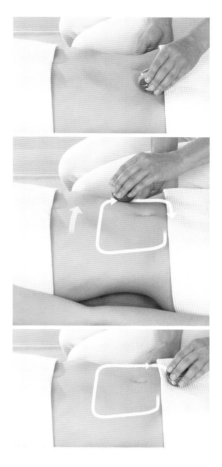

Massage the entire tummy with small, rolling movements with the crystal sphere, about three times along the course of the large intestine. Please be very sensitive and empathetic; observe where the movement of the sphere appears to be more pleasant or less pleasant for your partner and vary the pressure accordingly. It is generally better to ease up on the pressure in the area of the bladder.

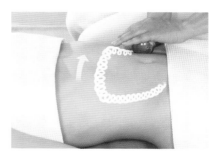

In order to render the tummy area really free, and as a happy ending, so to speak, begin at the navel and move in dynamic but light movements several times in a spiral, circling movement, clockwise, across the stomach.

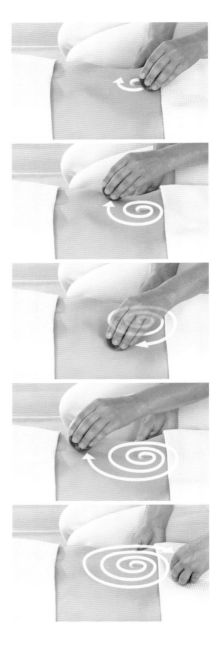

Now draw the sphere away from the body, as if also intentionally taking away anything that is burdening the person, and then lay aside the sphere.

Afterwards, stroke the tummy outward with your hands, as if you were intending to open it up to receive everything that is beautiful in life.

Then use your hands again to move across the tummy gently, in the way in which you would do yourself when you have eaten something particularly enjoyable.

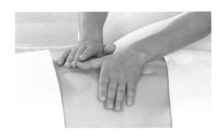

Depending on whatever impulse comes to you, choose a suitable palmstone crystal (I usually go for the Orange Calcite) and briefly lay it on the navel to fill up the tummy with sunlight and warmth.

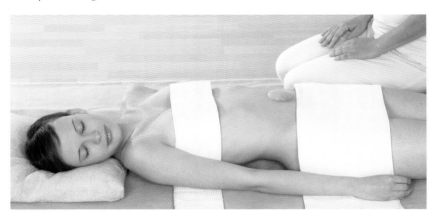

Back on your feet

In order to get your partner 'back on her feet' again, massage once more along the legs with the crystal spheres or the palm-stone crystals. Work with one or two crystals, treating either one leg after the other, or, if you only have a little time at your disposal, work on both legs at the same time. During this massage, you will once again connect with the detox meridians, especially of the bladder, kidneys, liver and gall bladder, so that, right at the end, the act of 'letting go' is stimulated again in every respect.

On the upper sides of the thighs, allow the palmstone crystals to glide parallel from the knee upward, and then draw them, to the right and left, along the side, into the back of the knees. Repeat this movement about three times.

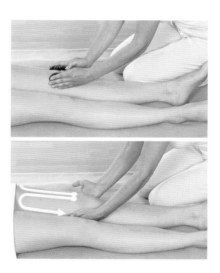

Circle around the knee from all sides (Amber is the first choice of crystal for knee joint problems).

Then, with the palmstone crystals, starting to the right and left of the ankles, glide along the upper side of the calf to the knee, then back, pulling on both sides to the tips of the toes.

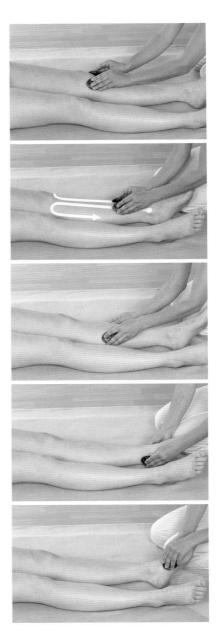

Draw the palmstone crystals from the thighs along the sides to the tips of the toes, one along each side of the leg. If you like, you can imagine that, as you are stroking downwards, all those things that are no longer of any use to your partner are leaving her body, while at the same time fresh energy is flowing in.

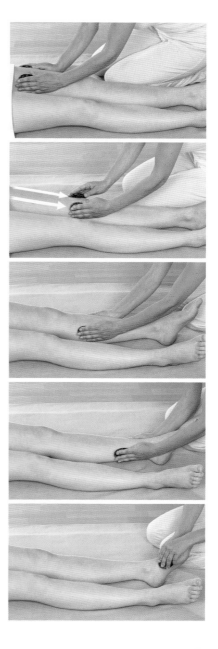

Gently knead the whole leg from the ankle, upward, and back with flowing movements.

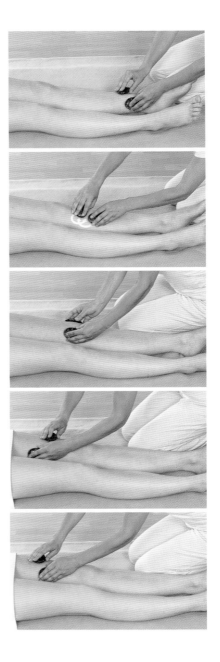

Afterwards, circle around the ankle bones.

Then draw outward from the ankle bones to the toes.

At the end, once again stroke the legs in long movements, using your hands.

Encircle the backs of both feet with your hands and gently pull.

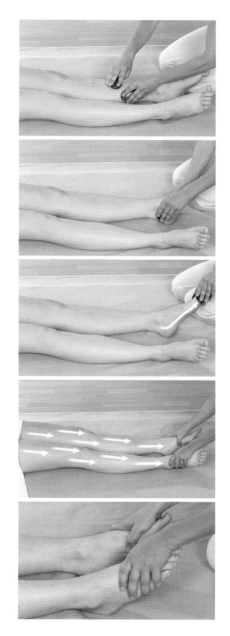

Then, right at the end, securely hold both heels in your hands. During a particularly intense treatment session, you may have become so involved with the massage that your energy has become intermingled with that of your massage partner. In which case, now is the time to draw back and separate your energies again. You may also like to say a little mental 'thank you'. It is a gift to receive a massage, but the trust of those who submit to it is also worthy of thanks.

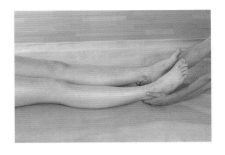

Allow your massage partner to rest for a while, covered up, and take a closer look at her. Maybe she has a little smile on her lips, which was not there before, or the facial muscles are visibly more relaxed, and the network of little wrinkles is less pronounced than before. Maybe your partner will get up from the treatment with a realization and sense of her own beauty that she would not have had without the massage. Doesn't she really look 'more beautiful'? This is really what the Crystal Balance is all about: to awaken that inner personal beauty and bring it out into the open. It is intended to reawaken that love of one's self and to activate self-healing energies. The effects of the crystals in combination with intense physical contact never cease to amaze me. I wish you much joy and pleasure with trying it out, and you will see that you, too, as the person giving the treatment will feel more balanced afterwards, just as the person receiving it.

It is very important to offer your massage partner something to drink after the treatment and to point out to her that she should drink at least two to three litres of still water a day during the next few days (we should always do this, anyway, but...). Depending on which crystal you have worked with, the Crystal Balance may visibly support the detoxification of the body; thus, if too little fluid is taken your partner may feel unwell or experience headaches – the so-called 'toxic headache'.

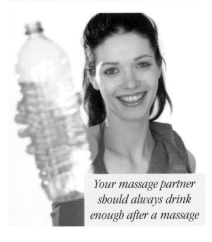

Your massage partner should always drink enough after a massage

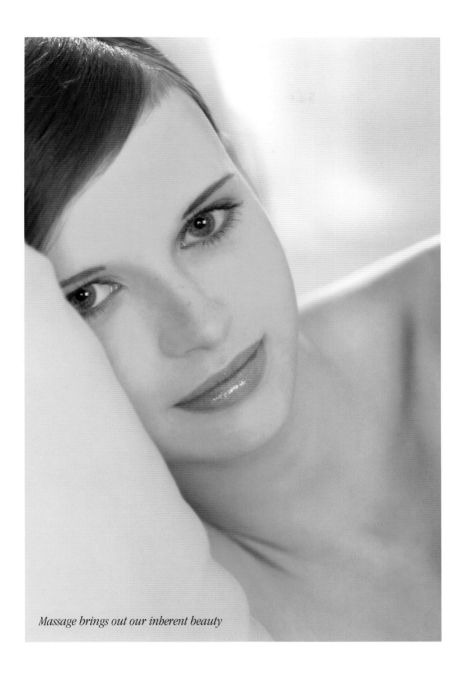

Massage brings out our inherent beauty

Crystals for beauty –
the facts

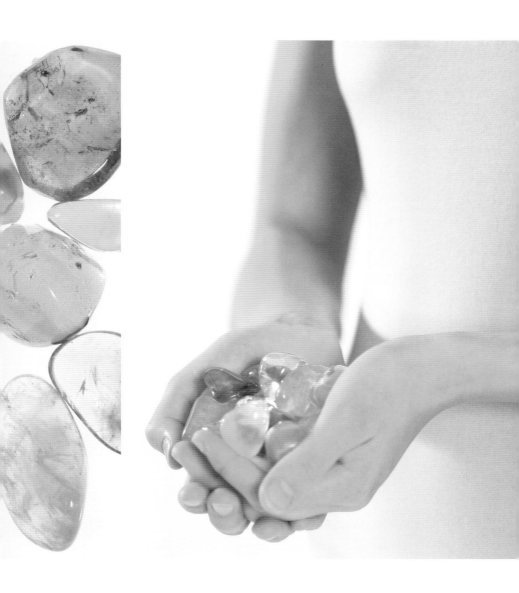

The aim of Crystal Balance

The aim of Crystal Balance is to create beauty through hands-on treatment and relaxation. Of course, the use of the crystals during the massage can and will, in addition, bestow positive effects on the physical, mental and spiritual levels. This can also be encouraged through wearing the crystals in question after the massage.

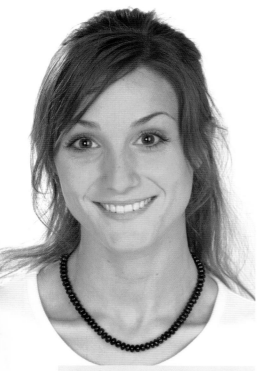

Extending and deepening the effects of the massage through wearing the crystals afterwards

Changes in the skin, reddening, pimples, allergies and other types of manifestations of the skin show us that the body is out of balance. Thus, for example, problems with the digestion often manifest as eruptions around the mouth area. The following extract from a text on Chinese medicine shows how general changes in the skin can be viewed in another light:

> 'What the kidneys do not eliminate is eliminated by the intestine.
>
> What the intestine does not eliminate is eliminated by the skin.
>
> What the skin does not eliminate will kill us.'

A real challenge for me as a natural beauty therapist is to get to the bottom of any skin problem that lasts for a considerable amount of time. There is a wonderful opportunity for using the crystals to support this harmonization process. The following crystals in particular have proven to be effective for beauty care and for use in Crystal Balance. You will find further properties and uses of crystals for the body, mind and spirit in the literature section in the appendix.

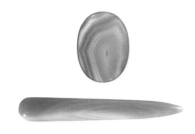

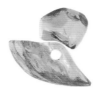

Amber

Amber is extremely effective as a warm amber-oil massage and it works positively on the joints, helps lift moods and provides a real sense of inner wellbeing. As a wound-healing resin from trees, it provides elasticity as well as protection in cases of dry, irritated skin.

Agate

Agate helps you feel comfortable in your own skin. It protects and supports you when you feel out of sorts. Its distinctive bands and layers correspond to the different layers in our own skin. As a result it is particularly effective at harmonizing and resolving a number of dermatological problems.

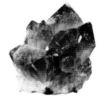

Amethyst

Amethyst is particularly effective at purifying and cleansing the skin, and combating reddening. It is very good for making face tonics for use on skin impurities and rosacea and also good for the intestines. If you are suffering from a tension headache, stroke the affected area of the head with an Amethyst druse to help relieve it (see Michael Gienger, *The Healing Crystal First Aid Manual* published by Earthdancer, a Findhorn Press Imprint). Massaging the

Amazonite

Its positive effect on the autonomic nervous system also helps with skin conditions caused by nervous problems (they are far more common than you might think!). Amazonite balances mood swings and has a calming effect.

soles of the feet with an Amethyst druse is extremely pleasant. Cleanse the energies of healing crystals by placing them on an Amethyst druse (see the section on Cleansing and Care, page 102).

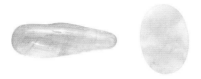

Aquamarine

This works quickly to combat streaming eyes. Massage the eyes gently with cool tumbled Aquamarine or use an eye compress moistened with Aquamarine gem water. Aquamarine helps combat allergic reactions in the skin, the mucous membranes and the respiratory system (for example with hay fever). It also relaxes the facial features.

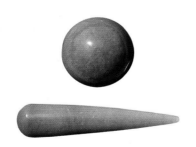

Aventurine

Aventurine combats inflammation and is ideal for skin eruptions and allergies. It strengthens the connective tissues and relieves pain. It is effective for sunburn and sunstroke, particularly in conjunction with Prase.

Tip: Today fewer people spend hours sunbathing, but sunburn or sunstroke suffered when walking or on holiday can be relieved by drinking Prase or Aventurine water. Put the crystals in a carafe of water for a few hours and then take regular sips. Aventurine water is extremely effective when used as a facial toner, freshly prepared on a regular basis.

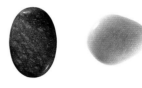

Blue Quartz

Blue Quartz lowers blood pressure and has cooling and soothing effects, making it the ideal crystal for people who are highly agitated and stressed. Blue Quartz has a calming and relaxing effect.

Note: At an exhibition, I gave a Blue Quartz crystal to a woman who was very nervous, had problems sleeping and was unable to relax properly. Shortly afterwards, she called me in an anxious state to say that she had treated one of her own clients with crystals, and the client had fainted. As I spoke to her it became clear that she had enthusiastically tried out the Blue Quartz meant for her on an exhausted client with low blood pressure. This demonstrates just how powerful crystals can be! However, since using them herself she has slept really well.

Calcite, orange

Generally, Calcite has a very stabilizing effect, while the beautiful blue variety tends to stimulate and balance the lymph flow. The yellow-orange variety is vitalizing and uplifting. It has a positive effect on the formation and development of bones. It is also excellent for massaging children. In addition, the Orange Calcite is very well suited for the 'warm sun in your tummy' aspect of Crystal Balance.

Chalcedony, blue

This crystal helps eliminate water retention (oedema), acting as a powerful stimulant on the lymph flow. It helps to expel dissolved toxins. I like to use this crystal for lymph drainage, especially on the lymph glands in the neck. Chalcedony is also good for detoxifying.

Chrysocolla

This is one of the typical anti-stress crystals; it balances mood swings and helps you keep a cool head. When used to massage the lower back it is effective for menstrual problems. It stimulates the regeneration of tissue, thereby helping to heal burns and scars. It is also effective for tense muscles and tissues in which toxins have become deposited.

Chrysoprase

This crystal dissolves toxins from the tissues and eliminates them via the lymph channels. It is one of the most effective detoxifying crystals, and it is also helpful for treating fungal infections and neurodermatis.

Citrine

Unfortunately, genuine Citrine is not cheap and is also hard to find as a sphere. However, it is particularly effective at lifting moods, reawakening inner happiness and combating feelings of depression. It is also used successfully in an Aurum Manus® massage for treating tinnitus and migraines.

Dumortierite

This is known as the 'take-it-easy' crystal, so-called because it calms the nervous system, helps with headaches caused by metabolic disturbances and works on skin problems and emotional upsets. It is a powerful crystal when used as a support during addiction recovery. It induces feelings of relaxation and contentment.

Emerald

Emerald is an 'all round health-giving crystal', and even Hildegard von Bingen said it could heal all the complaints that plagued humans. Emerald helps with inflammations of all kinds, especially in connection with intestinal and respiratory complaints, and is also effective on skin problems linked with these. Emerald has a detoxifying effect, fortifies the liver and stabilizes the nerves; it also helps alleviate feelings of fuzziness in the head (as if slight pressure were being exerted on it, similar to the sensation caused by a rather tight hat), headache or neck ache and even epilepsy and other disturbances in brain function. It is particularly helpful for people seeking a new direction in life.

Epidote

The body needs to regenerate immediately following an illness or after a period of time during which the body has been drained of energy. Epidote is one of the most powerful crystals for convalescence. It speeds up the healing process, rebuilds and strengthens. After a massage, I like to supply the client with a crystal as a pendant on a chain to take home.

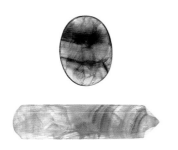

Fluorite

I use this crystal to massage clients who want to regain control of their lives, especially wives and mothers looking to 'find themselves' again. It also helps with chronic tension and with allergies that can often arise. It is one of the best 'learning crystals', and because clients frequently come for a Crystal Balance session before an exam, it is my first choice for such a massage. I often give them a piece of tumbled crystal or a pendant to take home.

Halite

When worn about the body, this transparent, cubic crystal salt helps to process electro-smog. It also helps reduce headaches and banish worries. When moistened and then passed over the forehead and neck, Halite can improve the distribution of energy in the body, and it protects and purifies the energy field. It also improves the general appearance of the skin. When using Halite in a massage, make sure you grind it finely and mix with oil, or choose a piece with a completely even surface.

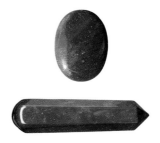

Heliotrope

What echinacea is to healing with plants, Heliotrope is to crystal healing. It strengthens the immune system and is effective in massages if your massage partner feels she is catching a cold or something similar.

Used *at the correct time* it may support the immune system and act as an anti-inflammatory. I have also found that it is effective if worn for several days after a massage.

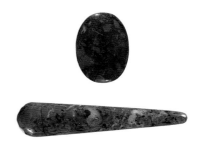

Hematite

I rarely use this crystal for massage because it has a particularly powerful stimulating effect due to its very high iron component, and my clients generally need peace and recovery rather than stimulation. However, it can be employed quite effectively in massages to awaken the inner spirit. It should not be used for inflammations, as it would exacerbate them. You should also be aware that evening massages can be too stimulating, leaving the person ready for action rather than sleep.

Jasper, red

With its iron content and distinctive red colouring, Jasper resembles Hematite, but is a little gentler. A massage with Red Jasper helps you tackle tasks with energy and enthusiasm. In winter, in particular, it has a wonderfully warming effect and helps to overcome prolonged feelings of weakness and tiredness. However, it is not suitable for those of nervous or heated dispositions, as they would probably leap up from the massage couch and head off at speed …

Kabamba Jasper

Kabamba Jasper is a relatively new crystal, extremely effective at opening up the pores and thereby encouraging detoxification through perspiration. It is good to use before a sauna or to assist when total body detox treatments are to be employed. The most recent research suggests that it has an immune-strengthening effect, especially for flu epidemics.

Magnesite

With its magnesium content, this crystal is used for deep relaxation, stress reduction and the prevention of cramp in the calves. It also combats rosacea and is good for angry red patches and other reddening of the skin. It encourages relaxation of the muscles and combats nervousness and stress.

Malachite

This crystal is used for all forms of cramp. It is especially helpful for complaints in the pelvic area and for menstrual problems. In addition, Malachite encourages sensuality and a desire for adventure. It also helps release unexpressed, pent-up feelings, and you need to bear this in mind during a massage. Any negative comments and minor complaints you may hear are unlikely to be directed against the person giving the massage, but are simply ways of 'letting off steam' and indications of a process of emotional cleansing. Malachite also has a physically purifying effect and is therefore good for rheumatic complaints.

Mookaite

This crystal brings spiritual balance, strengthens the immune system, provides a steady energy and encourages purification of the blood. It is an outstanding crystal for the spleen and for bringing harmony to the stomach organs. Mookaite helps to keep us centred and maintain a balance between our outer activity and inner calm. It is a balancing crystal – especially when used during a Crystal Balance treatment!

Moonstone

Moonstone is *the* crystal to use for conditions resulting from hormonal changes. This is especially the case for girls and women during puberty, menstruation and the menopause, or after giving birth. Moonstone also regulates the hormones of other glands, thereby improving the quality of sleep, for example, and helping with sleepwalking if used during a new moon and worn constantly for an entire moon cycle.

This crystal's connection with the moon is particularly evident in massage. It is much more stimulating around the time of the full moon than at a new moon. The different qualities of the various moon phases, are particularly apparent with the use of Moonstone. It also strengthens powers of intuition and empathy.

Moss Agate

On a spiritual level, Moss Agate relieves feelings of weight, pressure and emotional burden. Since these emotions are often felt 'on the chest', it is my favourite crystal for use during a 'Feel Free' Crystal Balance treatment on the upper chest area. Moss Agate is used during crystal healing because of its dissolving or loosening effect, and is often employed for coughs and colds, which often manifest in the chest area.

Nephrite

This crystal is particularly effective on the bladder, kidneys — the body's 'waterworks'. As a green crystal, it also helps to detoxify and strengthen the liver, or unblock it. In China it has long been used for balancing yin and yang. It seems to have a harmonizing effect, by stimulating those who are lethargic or calming down those who are overexcited. For example, it may give a lazy person a proverbial 'kick in the pants' and the impetus to act but equally allow the workaholic to feel able to take a holiday. Nephrite first supplies the necessary balance and later introduces a deeper equilibrium, a harmony between peace and activity. In our times of extremes, Nephrite is an important healing crystal.

 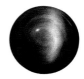

Obsidian

Obsidian improves blood circulation and energy supply to cool and numb parts of the body. It helps heal cellular disorders and gives relief from shocks and old traumas. As a result, it is a good crystal to use for persistent pain or sluggish healing. It is a volcanic glass and as such can be very stimulating. You should use it briefly, but also repeatedly, in massage.

because it stimulates the metabolism. It is worth trying out in cases of excess weight caused by a lack of 'grounding'.

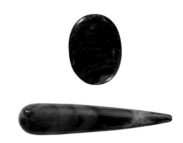

Ocean Agate (Ocean Jasper)

This crystal tones the tissues, encourages lymph flow and detoxification and stabilizes the immune system. It encourages cellular regeneration and can, therefore, be effective with cysts and tumours as it helps hinder growth. It can also be used for all degenerative skin complaints.

Prase

This crystal is excellent for treating swellings, skin irritations and reddening, especially after sunburn. In order to treat like with like, the crystal should be warmed slightly before use in treatment. It also has a calming, harmonizing effect.

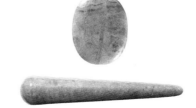

Petrified Wood

This is particularly good for people who 'don't have both feet on the ground', so to speak. It helps bring them back down to earth and to place their feet firmly back on the ground once more. I also like to massage the stomach area with Petrified Wood

Rhodonite

This 'first aid' crystal helps the skin heal after acne treatment and when supported by Black Tourmaline it is effective at healing scars by stimulating the regeneration of new cells.

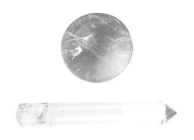

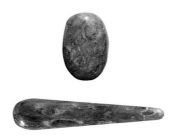

Rock Crystal

Rock Crystal firms up the skin and connective tissue, energizes and refreshes both body and spirit, and brings new vitality and clarity. Its efficacy is increased when used on a face mask. At the end of my treatment, I like to place a Rock Crystal on the 'third eye' (the point between the eyebrows) for a few minutes.

Ruby-Kyanite-Fuchsite

This crystal combines three minerals, which makes it particularly interesting for massage. It helps with stress by dissolving tension and brings relaxation coupled with the necessary strength but without excessive stimulation. Positive results have been noted on some heart problems, as well as with narrowing of blood vessels. However, when used in massage, Ruby-Kyanite-Fuchsite has proven to be particularly effective on stubborn back complaints especially in the lower back area and on the lumbar vertebrae.

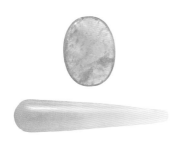

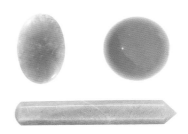

Rose Quartz

The skin really does look 'rosy' after a massage with Rose Quartz! It promotes gentle blood circulation and is one of the best introductory crystals for Crystal Balance, due to its vitalizing and rejuvenating effect. It is a good crystal for general indulgence and pampering.

Serpentine

This crystal encourages commitment and dedication, but also brings a sense of protection. It balances excessive acid, helps with nervousness and stress, brings a sense of peace and helps combat negative energetic influences. It is one of the crystals I use most in massage.

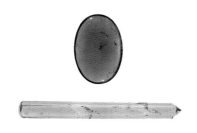

Smoky Quartz

On the one hand this crystal helps us cope better with problems and worries and on the other it dissolves tension. Smoky Quartz is particularly effective at treating extreme tension in the muscles of the back and the jaw. I have also had much success by giving my client two large tumbled crystals to hold during the treatment.

Sodalite

Sodalite has a similar effect to Blue Quartz, and is cooling and calming. It also encourages the body's ability to absorb fluids and is thus a very interesting crystal for problems with dry skin. Care should be taken with people who have low blood pressure.

Sunstone

The name of this crystal reflects its properties. It allows us to perceive the brighter, more positive aspects of life and helps us adopt a life-affirming and joyful attitude – to discover our own personal sun, as it were. Sunstone has a harmonizing effect on the autonomic nervous system and is one of the best crystals to use for depression. It is a wonderful crystal but is hard to find as a sphere. A massage can be carried out with a large tumbled crystal (which are unfortunately also quite rare).

Tiger Iron

Tiger Iron is a Hematite-Jasper-Tiger Eye mineral and harmonizes the various effects of these minerals. Like all gems that contain iron as a mineral substance, it has an enlivening and dynamic effect. The iron content is helpful with pale skin and dark rings under the eyes if these occur through a lack of iron in the blood. In addition, gems containing iron encourage the absorption of oxygen into the blood. It is important to watch out for signs of nervousness, excessive energy and lack of sleep and to stop using the crystal if these occur.

Topaz

This is a very beautiful crystal which promotes self-confidence, strengthens our abilities and has a positive effect on the nerves. It is extremely expensive, making it almost impossible to find as a sphere, palmstone or rod. Care should be taken with dark blue Topaz, as it is usually irradiated. The bluer the colour, the more likely it is to have been 'treated' in such a way. The natural blue of Topaz is never darker than sky-blue.

Tourmaline, black (Schorl)

I find that the positive effect Black Tourmaline has on neural conductivity makes it one of the best crystals for healing scars. The older the scars, the longer the healing takes, so I always advise placing small

Tourmaline rods in the direction of the flow of the relevant energy meridians at the earliest opportunity and then to massage with the crystal as well. It is also one of the best and most protective crystals, particularly against unwanted external influences, as well as radiation damage, which, unfortunately, almost always shows up in my tests. Wearing this crystal may at least provide some relief if you try, at the same time, to keep the radiation stress (from mobiles, digital cordless phones, etc.) to a minimum. After massaging with a Schorl crystal I always sense that a missing protective layer has been replaced. A total body treatment using small Black Tourmaline rods is also interesting to perform and encourages the flow of energy.

Tourmaline, green (Verdelite)

Practically unobtainable as a sphere, palmstone or rod, Green Tourmaline is still an important detoxifying crystal. It encourages the flow of energy and neural conductivity and is also particularly effective when used to help heal scars.

Tourmalinated Quartz

Minuscule needles of Schorl embedded within the quartz are a feature of Tourmalinated Quartz, especially in Rock Crystal or in Milk Quartz. The effect is similar to that of Schorl. In addition, it connects forces in life that are apparently contradictory (light and dark) and strengthens the nerves.

Zoisite with Ruby

This crystal is a powerful regenerator and its Ruby content also lends strength and the courage to make a new start. Its components are even more dynamic than those of Epidote. Zoisite with Ruby also strengthens fertility and potency, so I recommend that partners massage each other with this crystal when required. I believe it is always worth trying, and crystal massage does, after all, promote feelings of togetherness and harmony!

Cleansing and care

The rods, palmstones and spheres used in Crystal Balance should be cleansed thoroughly after each massage. First remove the remnants of the massage oils and rub the gems dry. Try using the Amethyst-Frankincense Cleansing Lotion, which removes almost all traces of the energies absorbed during the massage by the crystal/s. It can also be used to cleanse the body too and makes an excellent shower lotion.

Next, the crystals should be cleansed of the energies and information they have absorbed during the massage. For this purpose, hold the crystals under running water for a minute or longer and rub them vigorously with the fingers. You will find that the surfaces of the crystals, which will often feel a little 'soapy' at first, are more resistant after a while, and the fingers do not glide over them so easily. This indicates that absorbed energies have been removed.

Remove the crystals from the water and place them on an Amethyst druse. The Amethyst will free the crystals of any remaining 'foreign' information picked up from your massage partner and, a few hours later, the massage crystal will be 'fresh and new' again.

Store your massage crystals with care. A glass cabinet is ideal. Alternatively, wrap them in soft fabric and keep them in small, lined boxes – shops selling crystals sometimes pack them in suitable boxes. Although crystals may often appear 'lifeless'

to our eyes, I make a point of treating them like good friends and helpers, for whose effects and support I am very grateful. Many of the crystals with which I have worked in a spirit of 'cooperation' actually become clearer and more beautiful – something that has also been noted by my clients and by other people. Perhaps the gain in beauty is a mutual affair and what is given is also received. In any case, I enjoy their beauty and the beauty that, thanks to them, I see blossoming and unfolding under my hands time and again. I hope the readers of this book will have similar experiences with crystals and Crystal Balance. I bid you farewell with a traditional Native American greeting,

'Walk your path in beauty!'

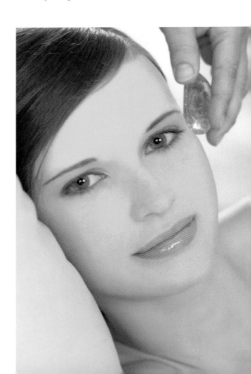

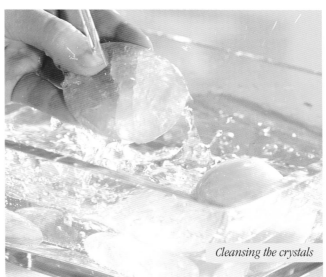

Cleansing the crystals

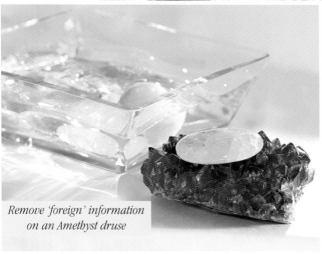

*Remove 'foreign' information
on an Amethyst druse*

The author

Even as a child, Monika Grundmann wanted to be a massage therapist. However, after leaving school she fell into an office job and belatedly completed her beauty therapy course while working. She soon realised that her interest lay not just in the physical, but in all aspects of the body – the person as a whole. She studied psychophysiognomy and completed her training as a non-medical practitioner. As a result of her training in the use of cosmetics Monika Grundmann was already very experienced in the power of touch, but she was now searching for a way to use touch as a positive influence on the whole person. She looked at Shiatsu, aromatherapy massage, Bach flower remedies, colour and sound treatments, and other areas, but training in crystal therapy with Michael Gienger finally brought her a better understanding of gems and their healing properties. She then began incorporating crystals in her own treatments in various ways.

Even before the birth of her daughter in 1999, she had been formulating a way to use crystals to improve the wellbeing of her clients and had already been encouraging Michael Gienger to write a book on the subject. However, the time was not yet right. In her search for a way to combine the techniques she had learned in a more focused,

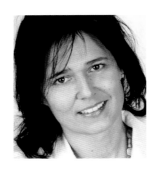

practical way, Monika Grundmann undertook training in 'Individual Therapy' with Rainer Strebel, which helped her discover the final piece of the jigsaw. The concept of 'Crystal Balance' was now complete. Inspired by the book, *Crystal Massage for Health and Healing* (published by Earthdancer an imprint of Findhorn Press in 2006), she felt it was now time to pass on all her tried and tested knowledge. This book is a culmination of the ten years she spent developing the concept, which she also now shares with others in seminars and training courses.

Acknowledgements

I would like to express my heartfelt thanks to all those who supported me while I was working on this book. Thanks to Michael Gienger for his committed support along the way as publisher, editor, picture editor, friend and patient teacher. Thanks also go to Walter von Holst for all those long, late-night telephone discussions and for sharing his experiences with crystal healing. Thanks to Ines Blersch for her outstanding photographs, the artistic concept and her ability to set beauty in the right light; also to Jens Volle for all his tireless and attentive co-operation in the photo studio; to Alexandra for her patience with the long hours of photo sessions and to Stefan Fischer of Fischercasting, Stuttgart, for finding Alexandra. I would also like to thank Laurin's Garten in Balingen, Peter Lind and Bea Diederich in Idar-Oberstein; the 'Kristall-shop Stuttgart' and the Marco Schreier mineral trading company in Ludwigsburg for the beautiful massage crystals; Ricky Welch for the Aurum Manus® massage; and Hans Halsbeck for the meticulous dowsing tests performed on my crystal massage oils, as well as Farfalla in Uster (Switzerland) for preparing the oils for me. I would like to thank Erwin Engelhardt for his advice on cleansing crystals, and especially on frankincense essential oil.

Very special thanks go to Fred Hageneder for all his graphic work, as well as for combining the photos and text into a successful layout, and of course I would also like to thank Andreas Lentz, my publisher, for making this book possible in the first place. Crystal Balance could never have been created without my teachers, whom I have to thank for my knowledge about massage and my holistic knowledge of humankind; thanks also to my clients and creative students, who have all contributed to the development of Crystal Balance. Thank you to Birgit Morrison, who spent many evenings with me as my massage partner and kept encouraging me to continue on my path. Finally, and with all my heart, I thank my mother, who quietly and gently supported me all the time, made the impossible possible and was always there for me when I needed someone most. This book was written for all of them and for my daughter, Paula. For us all I wish that physical contact might become an integral part of our lives again and that we will allow ourselves to be touched by Life.

Monika Grundmann
Heilsbronn, Spring 2006

Addresses

Crystal Balance
Monika Grundmann

Introductory courses, seminars and training in Crystal Balance, Crystal Sound Massage, Crystal Beauty and various other kinds of crystal massage can be booked directly with the author, as well as weekend introductory courses in crystal healing and dowsing.

At present, the seminars are available in Germany and Switzerland. It is possible to arrange international bookings.
International training in Crystal Balance with Monika Grundmann in English is planned. Information about dates and venues can be found on: www.crystal-balance.com

Introductory courses, seminars, training and materials for working with Crystal Balance and wholesale and retail suppliers:

Ausbildungs-Institut und Praxis
für Edelstein-Massagen und
Edelstein-Kosmetik
Edelstein-Balance®
Monika Grundmann
Bauhofstr. 14
91560 Heilsbronn
Germany
tel +49 (0)9872 - 2999
fax +49 (0)9872 - 2606
www.crystal-balance.com

EDELSTEIN
BALANCE
MONIKA GRUNDMANN

Suppliers

Suppliers of the Crystal Balance work trolley, Amethyst-Frankincense Cleansing Lotion and other accessories for Crystal Balance can be found on:
www.crystal-balance.com

Crystal Balance Oil manufacturer

Farfalla Essentials A.G.
Florastr. 18
8610 Uster
Schwitzerland
tel +41 -44-905 99 00
fax +41-44-905 99 09
www.farfalla-essentials.com
info@farfalla.ch

International distributors of
Crystal Balance Oils

US and Canada:
www.naturaleurope.com

All other countries:
www.crystal-balance.com

Further seminars and training

Reflexology with crystals

Institute, practitioners, lectures, seminars and training in reflexology and with crystal rods.

Ewald Kliegel
Rotenbergstrasse 154
70190 Stuttgart
Germany
www.reflex-zonen.de
info@reflex-zonen.de

Crystal massage and crystal healing

Consultations, seminars, basic and advanced training in crystal healing, crystal massage and related fields.

www.cairn-elen.de
info@cairn-elen.de

Non profit organisation for research and application of crystal healing:

Steinheilkunde e.V.
www.steinheilkunde-ev.de

More on crystal healing can be found on:
www.steinheilkunde.de

More useful addresses, which were not available at printing, can be found on:
www.crystal-balance.com

Bibliography

Michael Gienger, *The Healing Crystal First Aid Manual, A practical A to Z of common ailments and illnesses and how they can be best treated with crystal therapy,* published by Earthdancer, a Findhorn Press Imprint, in 2006

Michael Gienger, *Crystal Power Crystal Healing,* published by Cassell Illustrated in 1998

Michael Gienger, *Healing Crystals, The A-Z Guide to 430 Gemstones,* published by Earthdancer, a Findhorn Press Imprint, in 2005

Michael Gienger, *Crystal Massage for health and healing,* published by Earthdancer, a Findhorn Press Imprint, in 2006

Michael Gienger, *Gem Water, How to prepare and use more than 130 crystal waters for therapeutic treatments,* published by Earthdancer, a Findhorn Press Imprint, in 2008

This book introduces a spectrum of massage possibilities using healing crystals. The techniques have been developed and refined by experts, and this wisdom is conveyed in simple and direct language, enhanced by photos. Any interested amateur will be amazed at the wealth of new therapeutic possibilities that open up when employing the healing power of crystals.

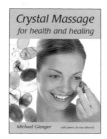

Michael Gienger
Crystal Massage for Health and Healing
112 pages, full colour throughout
ISBN 978-1-84409-077-8

All the important information about 430 healing gemstones in a neat pocket-book! Michael Gienger, known for his popular introductory work 'Crystal Power, Crystal Healing', here presents a comprehensive directory of all the gemstones currently in use. In a clear, concise and precise style, with pictures accompanying the text, the author describes the characteristics and healing functions of each crystal.

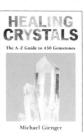

Michael Gienger
Healing Crystals
The A - Z Guide to 430 Gemstones
Paperback, 96 pages
ISBN 978-1-84409-067-9

This is an easy-to-use A-Z guide for treating many common ailments and illnesses with the help of crystal therapy. It includes a comprehensive colour appendix with photographs and short descriptions of each gemstone recommended.

Michael Gienger
The Healing Crystal First Aid Manual
A Practical A to Z of Common Ailments and Illnesses and How They Can Be Best Treated with Crystal Therapy
288 pages, with 16 colour plates
ISBN 978-1-84409-084-6

OTHER BOOKS BY EARTHDANCER

Adding crystals to water is both visually appealing and healthy. The water becomes infused with crystalline energy. It is a known fact that water carries mineral information and Gem Water provides effective remedies, acting quickly on a physical level. It is similar and complementary to wearing crystals, but the effects are not necessarily the same.

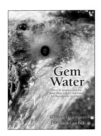

This book explains everything you need to know in order to begin preparing and using Gem Water, and provides important information on which crystals to use and which to avoid. The concept may appear simple at first, but you need to apply it with care, and the book explains all the facts you need to know before getting started.

Michael Gienger, Joachim Goebel
Gem Water
How to prepare and use more than 130 crystal waters for therapeutic treatments
Paperback, 96 pages, ISBN 978-1-84409-131-7

Using this guide the reader will discover which of the 360 crystal elements is associated with the position of the sun at the time of their birth; learn about the relationship between birth charts, crystals, and planets; and find out how personal crystal elements are connected to numerology. The book also explores Marc Edmund Jones's key words, Sabian symbols, and Jane Ridder-Patrick's healing body points, ultimately teaching the readers how to reach a higher life potential.

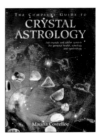

Marina Costelloe
The Complete Guide to Crystal Astrology
360 crystals and sabian symbols
for personal health, astrology and numerology
Paperback, 224 pages, full colour, with 360 images
ISBN 978-1-84409-103-4

Revealing the dynamic bond between man and tree, this inspired yoga handbook offers a detailed review of the ancient wisdom of Kundalini Yoga and unveils the inner power of trees, as well as their unique characteristics and energies. Yoga exercises based on this wisdom are provided, each of which operates by fostering a connection with the inner essence of a different tree, from birch and lime to elm and rowan. With full illustrations and step-by-step instructions.

Satya Singh, Fred Hageneder
Tree Yoga: A Workbook
Strengthen Your Personal Yoga Practice
Through the Living Wisdom of Trees
Paperback, two colours, 224 pages
ISBN 978-1-84409-119-5

There are two types of angels: those with wings, and those with leaves. For thousands of years, those seeking advice or wanting to give thanks to Mother Nature have walked the ancient paths into the sacred grove. Because today sacred groves have become scarcer, and venerable old trees in tranquil spots are hard to find when we need them, Earthdancer is pleased to present this tree oracle to bring the tree angels closer to us all once more.

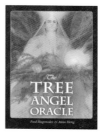

Fred Hageneder, Anne Heng
The Tree Angel Oracle
36 colour cards (95 x 133 mm), plus book, 112 pages
ISBN 978-1-84409-078-5

Crystal Balance
Monika Grundmann

First edition 2008

This English edition © 2008 Earthdancer GmbH
English translation © 2008 Astrid Mick
Editing of the translated text by JMS Books LLP

Originally published in German as *Schönheit durch Berühren*
World Copyright © Neue Erde GmbH, Saarbruecken, Germany
2006

Original German text copyright © Monika Grundmann 2006

Cover Photography: Ines Blersch
Cover Design: Dragon Design, GB

Photos: Ines Blersch, Stuttgart
Assistance: Jens Volle
Photo Model: Alexandra

Hair and Make-up: Petra Ucakar, Stuttgart
Casting: fishercasting.de, Stuttgart

Typesetting and graphics: Dragon Design UK
Typeset in Garamond Condensed

Printed and bound in China

ISBN 978-1-84409-132-4

Published by Earthdancer, an imprint of:
Findhorn Press, 305a The Park,
Forres, IV36 3TE, Scotland.
www.earthdancerbooks.com
www.findhornpress.com

For further information and book catalogue contact:
Findhorn Press, 305a The Park, Forres, IV36 3TE, Scotland.
Earthdancer Books is an imprint of Findhorn Press.

tel +44 (0)1309-690582   fax +44 (0)1309-690036
info@findhornpress.com   www.earthdancer.co.uk   www.findhornpress.com

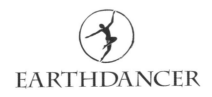

EARTHDANCER

A FINDHORN PRESS IMPRINT